# Diagnosis Male

# Diagnosis Male

## Troy Harvey

HarperCollins*Publishers*

For anyone suffering.
Get well soon.

**HarperCollins***Publishers*

First published in Australia in 2011
by HarperCollins*Publishers* Australia Pty Limited
ABN 36 009 913 517
harpercollins.com.au

**HarperCollins***Publishers*
Level 13, 201 Elizabeth Street, Sydney NSW 2000, Australia
31 View Road, Glenfield, Auckland 0627, New Zealand
A 53, Sector 57, Noida, UP, India
77–85 Fulham Palace Road, London, W6 8JB, United Kingdom
2 Bloor Street East, 20th floor, Toronto, Ontario M4W 1A8, Canada
10 East 53rd Street, New York NY 10022, USA

National Library of Australia Cataloguing-in-Publication data:

Harvey, Troy.
  Diagnosis male / Troy Harvey.
  ISBN: 978 0 7322 9259 1 (pbk.)
A823.4

Cover design: Katherine Hall, de Luxe & Associates
Cover photography: Alex Craig
Internal design by Alicia Freile, Tango Media
Typeset in 10/14pt Hoefler Text by Kirby Jones

# contents

# PREFACE

The human body is an amazing machine. Stop for a moment and imagine, if you can, the millions upon millions of tiny little parts, cells, tubes, germs, hairs and other paraphernalia, all working in perfect unison to keep you kicking along each day with little to worry about other than taxes and the possibility that someone will create another series of *Big Brother*. Every single part of your body is currently harmonising with every other single part of your body to ensure you don't just stop one day and keel over. It is such a major operation, such a fantastic construction, that it's hard to believe the human body keeps working as brilliantly as it does, as often as it does.

Of course, it also often doesn't.

The tiniest problem can set off a chain of events that will leave you emptying yourself from both ends, excreting sweat from every pore, gasping for air and wishing with all your heart that you hadn't touched that door handle in the men's toilets at the train station last week. And when those sorts of problems do present themselves, most men face a terrible decision: ride it out or go and see a doctor. But there really isn't much of a choice. Quite simply, real men don't go to doctors.

Now, in case it needs saying — and perhaps it might during the chapters that follow — let me state up-front that I am not a hypochondriac. Okay? According to common definition, a sufferer of hypochondria is convinced that they're ill despite having symptoms that are neither present nor likely. But I'm talking here about symptoms that *are* present. They are not perceived or a manifestation of an overactive imagination. Me, I'm just a regular guy who has an unnatural fear of dying and I'll do whatever it takes to avoid death for as long as possible. And yes, that might mean having to seek medical help occasionally.

Just so long as we're clear on that hypochondria thing ...

Anyway, being a man, there's a bit of a stigma attached to visiting a doctor. It can be seen as weak or unmanly to admit you have any sort of ailment, so most guys will ignore whatever illness it is they are suffering through and hope it simply disappears over time. Even in the event that an electric saw has slipped from his grasp and sliced through the wrist clear to the bone, there's a good chance your average male would just discard the limb and proceed with the task in front of him. Unless a woman is present, of course.

Frankly, in the above electric-saw misadventure, if there wasn't a rational-minded female around to spout the magic words 'Maybe you should go and see a doctor', most men would probably just figure, *Hey, I guess I'm left-handed now. I'd better start practising my new signature.* It's not really about machismo, nor any sort of embarrassment. It's more the simple fact that we're really lazy.

Going to the doctor is a hassle. It's a pain in the butt, and one that will probably go away if we ignore it. Women, on the other hand, will suggest visiting a doctor for the most minor of ailments. A basic sniffle of mine has often resulted in the following discussion with my beautiful partner:

'Honey, maybe you should go and see a doctor.'

'A doctor? Why?' I ask, pointlessly.

'Because I just heard you sniffle. It could be the start of something.'

'Or the end of a sniffle.'

'No, seriously — it's better to find out early on, before it sets in.'

'Before *what* sets in?'

'Well, it could be anything.'

'Like what?'

'Well, it could be influenza, sinus, hay fever, a deviated septum, inflamed lymph nodes, colon cancer, the black plague, scarlet fever, Scarlett Johansson fever, osteoporosis, acne, dengue fever, a trick knee, malaria, bird flu, scurvy ... or that weird thing Lou Gehrig had.'

'Lou Gehrig's disease?'

'Yeah, that's the one.'

'It's just a sniffle! I'll be fine.'

But inevitably they talk you into going to see a doctor, who, after making you wait for an eternity to ponder the possibility of all those possibilities, charges you $100 to tell you that it is, in fact, just a sniffle. Then the doctor has a joke with the nurses at your expense once you've left. (I'm sure of it.)

The other thing about guys and health is that we don't actually *have* doctors. Women do. Women have doctors who delivered them at birth and continue to treat them until they're old and grey. They know everything about each other and talk in front of you, if you happen to be present, like you're a third wheel. It's very awkward.

Personally, I have rarely been to the same doctor twice. There are two reasons for this. One, because I don't want another person knowing everything about me. I like to spread the information around. And two, because who has the energy and commitment to forge this kind of bond with another human being? I can barely keep a girlfriend; I certainly can't keep a doctor. I'm not there to make friends, all I want is someone to tell me the problem and that it can be fixed by taking something twice daily before meals. Keep it simple — I'm a guy.

I remember once when I was dating a girl and became slightly unwell for the first time in our relationship. 'Maybe you should go and see a doctor,' she suggested — to which I begrudgingly agreed. I made my disdain for such a notion quite obvious, however.

'Fine, I'll call him for you,' she said eventually. 'Do you have the number?'

'What number?'

'Your doctor's number.'

'Which doctor?'

'How many do you have?'

'None. I do all right financially but I don't keep anyone *on staff*, if that's what you're asking.'

'Well, who's your regular doctor, then?'

'Whoever's there at the medical centre.'

'Fine. And which medical centre do you go to?'

'Whichever is closest when I'm sick.'

At this point, she promptly lost her mind.

At the risk of repeating myself, if there isn't a woman nearby at the time of illness or injury to utter that wonderful phrase — 'Maybe you should go and see a doctor' — then guys probably won't even consider it.

Going to a doctor doesn't make sense to us. If it falls off, then we'll make do without it. If it makes us ill, we'll somehow soldier on. And if it kills us then, damn it, we'll just have to miss *The Simpsons*. All up, I can't help thinking that most doctors wouldn't have a job if it weren't for women.

Now, don't get me wrong, all you medical types out there, I'm all for what you do. I'm a huge fan. But, for the life of me, I can't imagine why anyone would choose to rummage around inside someone else's body or be near sick people for a living. Still, without doctors we'd all be dying a lot younger, I realise, and suffering through things we never want to be suffering through.

So thank you, doctors, for all your hard work. Personally though, if I never have to experience first-hand any more of this hard work of yours, I'd really appreciate it ...

And to my fellow men, if you do have a problem that needs to be checked out, then it's probably best to seek professional help as soon as possible. Going to the doctor can be embarrassing and hurt the ego a little, but it could be worth it to live a few extra hours. You never know when something cool is going to happen in life, and it would be terrible to miss it.

Having said all that, this book is about some of the times when a woman was present during one of my many illnesses or injuries, and therefore about the multitude of times I, as a man, have actually been to the doctor. And, quite possibly, why I may never, ever go back again as long as I live.

# 1
# THE BOTTOM LINE

No guy wants to tell a doctor that he has a problem with his backside. It is so far down the list of things men would ever choose to do that it's actually preceded by 'Buying tampons' and 'Talking about our feelings'.

There's some irony in this. A fair proportion of guys will drop their trousers at the drop of, well, a pair of trousers, to bare their arse to every stranger in a public place if the event calls for a mooning. They'll hang their naked cheeks out of a moving car for the world to see, if the lighting is right and the urge takes them. But ask one of those same blokes to show his back passage to a qualified medical professional and suddenly it's one of the most intimate acts that could ever take place. Personally, I'd rather exhibit my bum in a crowded museum than show it to one man with a torch and a lubricated finger, but sometimes you don't have a choice.

I'd been seeing a girl for almost two years when this situation occurred, so any discussion about my bottom wasn't too outrageous between us. Okay, so it wasn't the chosen topic over breakfast, but it wasn't taboo either. It's not like we were having conversations every morning along the lines of:

*'How's your muesli, darling?'*

*'It's all right. A little dry. How's your bum?'*

*'Oh, about the same — a little dry. How's yours?'*

*'Better than ever. I don't know why people go on about babies' bottoms so much — mine is so much more impressive. Smoother and more pleasant in photos.'*

That kind of thing just wasn't happening. But we were well past the awkward moments and open to talking about things that troubled us. Well, almost.

For some reason, I lowered my guard slightly too much one day and made the kind of comment that women long for while men question themselves for making for the rest of their lives. When you discuss such intimate matters, women think they're breaking down another barrier in the relationship. To me, conversations about bum trouble aren't barriers that need to be broken down. There are some things that could happily remain sacred. But there I was, early in the morning, and not thinking too clearly.

'Morning, honey,' my lovely partner remarked as I exited the bathroom. 'How are you today?'

'Fine,' I replied. 'Except, my bottom's a bit sore.'

Yikes! It just slipped out. Thank heavens I wasn't at the office when that little gem tripped from my lips. Imagine:

*'Morning, Troy. How are those reports going?'*

*'Oh fine. I'll have them on your desk by five, boss.'*

*'And the charts? Have you done the charts yet?'*

*'Still looking at them, sir. They're taking a bit of time. Between that and my sore arse, I'm really snowed under.'*

*'Your what?'*

*'My sore bottom, sir. I have a lot to do — charts, reports, dealing with a sore bum — deadlines are tight.'*

*'Troy, you might want to consider seeing a doctor.'*

*'What would a doctor know about these reports, boss?'*

*'Good point, Troy. Carry on.'*

Of course, when you admit to your partner that you're suffering from this kind of affliction, the resulting discussion is very, very different.

'Your bottom is sore?' she asked. 'What's wrong with it?'

'My ... um ... Oh, no, it's fine. I don't know why I said anything.'

'No, tell me. Why is it sore? It could be the start of something.'

'It isn't the start of anything. I shouldn't have mentioned it. Everything's fine.'

'Well, maybe you should go and see a doctor, just in case.'

And there they were. Those magic words. Sure, the conversation went on at length afterwards, during which swearwords were possibly muttered under my breath — but what was the point? When a woman utters that phrase, you're going to see a doctor whether you like it or not. But who would the lucky doctor be?

'I'll call Dr Smythe,' she announced. 'You saw him last time.'

'I don't like Dr Smythe,' I replied. 'He made me feel uneasy.'

'Uneasy? How?'

'He asked me if it hurt while he was prodding my stomach, and when it actually did hurt, he looked at me as if he *knew* it hurt — so I told him it didn't hurt, to prove him wrong. But I reckon he knew I was lying, so now I think he doesn't trust me.'

'Well, Troy, you were lying.'

'Yes, but he should've trusted me from the start.'

'But you *were lying*!'

'That's beside the point! My point is, he makes me feel uneasy and I'm not going to see him.'

'Fine. What about Dr Michaels? You saw him that time you had the sniffle.'

'Dr Michaels saw me in my old underpants and smirked.'

'He didn't smirk!'

'He smirked ... And his stethoscope was cold.'

'Well, what about Dr Rice?'

'Dr Rice is a woman! I don't want to show my butt to a woman!'

'I'm sure she's seen one before.'

'Not mine — and mine might be unique. You never know.'

'So who will you see?'

'Whoever's at the medical centre when I get there.'

These days, this final sentence is usually said in unison with my partner. She's almost reached the point of acceptance. Bless her.

So off I went to the medical centre closest to my apartment in the hope that the doctor on call that day was not only male but also one that had seen a bottom or two in his time. I'd have hated to surprise him.

A quick side note on proctologists — those men and women who have elected to practise a branch of medicine dealing solely with the rectum and the anus. For the life of me I cannot imagine why anyone would actually decide to make the arse their career. What kind of mindset does that take?

I mean, there they are at university with their colleagues, all of whom have chosen to study medicine, and the day comes when they're forced to pick the area they will specialise in for the rest of their lives. What goes through their heads during the selection process exactly?

*Hmmm, I could choose podiatry. But then again, would I want to deal with feet all day? Feet are so smelly and I'd hate to have to touch a stranger's foot region. No, that's not for me. What about surgery maybe? Let me think ... It seems fairly disgusting. You'd be covered in mess all the time. Mind you, I do like the rubber gloves ...*

So when they decide on the proctology route, they must be thinking purely about the money. And so they should!

Bless you, colon people. While I don't envy you one bit, I thank you. (I'd shake your hand, in fact, but ... well, you know.) Because I can't even imagine what your working day must be like, nor your average night at home for that matter ...

*'Hi honey, how was your day?'*

*'Oh, so so. Most of my clients today were just arseholes, but I did find some loose change up the back of old Mr Johnson.'*

*'Oh dear. Well, make sure you wash up before dinner. We're having bolognaise.'*

*'Er ... bolognaise ... Y'know, I might pass on that.'*

*'Really? Well, I made sticky date for dessert.'*

And so it goes.

Of course, the difference here is that these people have chosen to make a living out of the rectum. When someone walks into their practice, proctologists expect to see a person's arse. In fact, they encourage it. General practitioners — one of whom I was just about to see — are a different story altogether.

Imagine yourself to be a GP for just one moment. You're waiting for your next patient and it basically becomes a game of craps; you're rolling the dice, hoping for a win. Will they have hiccups or will you have to handle their wang? Will their eye need some drops or will their explosive diarrhoea haunt your nightmares for weeks to come? Who knows? You simply have to wait and see what will present itself when the patient's name is called.

And while I was thinking this, the next available doctor entered the waiting room and read a name off the list in front of him.

'Troy Harvey?'

*Snake eyes, doc! You lose.*

Just telling a GP you have bottom troubles isn't easy for a guy. The phrasing of this statement was something that had rattled about in my brain for quite some time. Bum issues, sore arse, crack rot, something not right with the back door ... what exactly do you say?

I decided to opt for the childish 'I have a sore bottom' — and instantly felt like a moron. You feel five years old when you speak those words aloud to a trained professional. And as soon as they slip out, you wish you'd just said 'hiccups' and been done with it.

'Well, we'd better take a look then,' the doctor replied without an air of concern.

'Sure,' I muttered. 'Uh ... I'm sorry.'

'Don't be. It happens all the time. Hop up on the table there on your hands and knees and we'll take a look.'

Now, I don't know if you've ever had someone look up your arse with a torch at close range before, but it's truly a unique experience. Warm, a little mysterious, and by far the only situation I never want to be in ever again so long as I stand on the face of this planet.

'Yep. It does seem to be a little chafed. I'll give you a cream for it,' said the doctor as though he'd seen it all before. And there I was thinking my backside was unique.

So I did up my pants and immediately regretted having been sent to the doctor's in the first place. Here I was, in the afterglow of one of the most humiliating experiences of my life (so far), being told that the condition I was experiencing would've cleared itself up over time — just as guys always assume it will. I needn't have come. I was *sent*.

The doctor handed me a prescription for a cream that, to this day, I've never bothered to pick up from the pharmacy. Why? Well, let me make this clear. If anyone reading this works for the manufacturer of a cream that heals rectal itches and pains, could you *please* not use the word 'anus' in the name of the product? It's a minor detail, but one for which almost all your customers would be eternally grateful.

The truth is, cute girls work in pharmacies. Sure, I'd most likely never see them again after picking up a prescription, but the fact that they're cute is enough to stop me purchasing anything that draws their attention to my damaged *anus*. End of story.

And for the record, my bum did get better all on its own. So keep the wise cracks to a minimum, people.

Okay, so *cracks* might not have been the best choice of words, but you get my point. Your turn will come.

# 2
# THE NIGHT I DIDN'T DIE OF A HEART ATTACK

At 3.12 on a random Tuesday morning some years back, I awoke suddenly with a searing, stabbing pain in my heart. It was as if a vindictive ex-girlfriend was performing voodoo on a small doll bearing my likeness. I could narrow it down to two possibilities, but as I hadn't seen either of them in several years, I felt it might be inappropriate to call at this hour and ask them to stop.

Slowly the pain subsided, though, and I reminded myself not to eat so close to bedtime in the future. I began the descent back to the land of slumber and saucy dreams, only to then be wrenched into reality once more with another stabbing sensation exactly where I assumed my heart was located. I'd seen it there on Valentine's Day cards, after all.

This activity continued throughout the morning until I decided to do something about it. I climbed out of bed, showered, and went to the office where I worked to see what others thought of my condition. Sensible, eh?

Over the course of the day I made loud mention of my impending doom, in the hope that my workmates would dismiss it as a mere heartburn or some sort of flu symptom. But this was not to be. A female colleague of mine, fed up with my moaning, decided to do some internet research and finally declared — without a shred of medical knowledge — that I should probably go and see a doctor. I quickly phoned my mother for a second opinion.

My mum, I believe, was once a nurse. Either that or she was just a big fan of *M\*A\*S\*H* when we were kids, I've never really been sure. I told her my problem and, in true motherly fashion, she completely overreacted and began dialling ooo on her other phone. I calmed her down with the promise that I would go to the medical centre immediately and have it checked out. And I did. (If by 'immediately' you mean four hours later, after work.)

The doctor was kind enough at first. A bit of gentle prodding and a few nonchalant questions later, however, and she was thrown into a ball of panic. So far I was the only calm person in this whole heart-condition fiasco.

After hastily scribbling a note on a formal-looking piece of paper, she jammed it into an envelope and advised me to phone a family member or friend and have them take me to the emergency department of the nearest hospital and give them the note. Right away.

This was all a bit serious, for two reasons. Firstly, because the only person who would be available was a girl I'd recently broken up with and I didn't wish to give her the satisfaction of thinking that she may have, literally, broken my heart. The other reason was that *The Simpsons* was on in twenty minutes. I hate to miss *The Simpsons*.

I ducked back home and set the timer on my video recorder before deciding to call on the most reliable person I knew to get me to the hospital. Myself. Of course, had I died on the way due to heart spasms, my reputation as a reliable guy who always comes through would've been shot to hell. But it was a risk I was willing to take.

I sped off to the emergency area, parked my car in the hospital's car park — which was the equivalent of three days' hard ride from the reception desk — and then made my way to the appropriate place. Seriously, it was a fifteen-minute walk from the car park to the emergency department. (That might need to be addressed; a man could have a heart attack walking that far.)

Inside the hospital's entrance I noticed a plethora of bleeding, screaming, crying and broken people waiting to be called up. I felt embarrassed, walking in with no visible signs of injury. They all looked at me with varying degrees of pity — because, as everyone knows, the serious cases are treated first in an emergency department, while anyone showing no visible signs would usually have to wait until sun-up.

Having handed the doctor's note to the nurse at the triage desk, I took a seat. She read it then quickly proceeded to show the note to five other nurses behind the desk. They gathered in a huddle, mumbling and occasionally pointing in my direction. Maybe they had heard about the sit-ups I'd been doing recently and were fighting over who would be the lucky one to see me with my shirt off.

Then, with the kind of urgency I have only ever seen in an episode of *ER*, all five nurses came running at me, demanded I sit in a wheelchair and, as a team, proceeded to ignore every other patient in the room and elevate me to celebrity status. What the hell did that note say?

Immediately after entering a side room, I was stripped to my underwear and questioned from every direction about my dietary and exercise habits. (Hey — I was naked. Could they not *see* I'd been doing sit-ups?) With even more vigour now, they soon began applying weird and exotic stickers all over my body.

The 'exotic' nature of the hospital sticker is one rarely described, but allow me to indulge in it for a moment. These stickers had press studs on them — that's right, the type of studs you find on ladies' chambray shirts or down the side of a male stripper's trousers. It seems I was about to die wearing the world's least fashionable combination: underpants and press-studded body stickers. The studs were connected via other press studs to wires that further connected to monitoring machines — which were (possibly) then connected to the mind of someone who knew what the hell all these wires, machines and press studs were for.

Moments before, I had been strolling through the main door of the emergency department feeling sorry for the obviously injured who were gathered there, waiting in agony. I hadn't even considered what might actually be wrong with me, the severity of the situation, or what would take place next. Now I was caught up in a whirlwind of activity and serious medical urgency.

I was advised by one of the nurses that they were running an ECG. If I'd actually known what that meant or even what 'ECG' stood for, I probably would've been quite concerned. But my ignorance served me well. Meanwhile, one of the other nurses continued to ask me about my eating habits.

'Terrible,' I responded.

She looked at the ECG printout and said, 'Well, perhaps this will serve as a wake-up call.'

I had a very good clock radio beside my bed at home, but this nurse probably didn't want to hear about that right now. She seemed far too engrossed in the reading material my heart had provided her.

With press-stud stickers still fastened to my body, I was then whisked through a series of tests and x-rays, scans and blood tests, questionnaires and probing, followed by more x-rays, scans, questions and blood tests. And then, after two hours of chaos and madness, I was placed on a bed and told to lie still and relax. As the word 'relax' came out of the doctor's mouth, a male nurse arrived with one of those machines you see in movies — you know, the one with electro-shock paddles attached, accompanied by some passionate medic yelling: '*Clear!*'

For a place that wanted me to relax, they really were doing a lot to make me very, very tense. A man could have a heart attack with this much excitement.

Then suddenly it was as if I was no longer the new toy in the playroom. Without warning, everyone left me to lie there, counting ceiling tiles and wondering whether I'd taped over something important when setting the video recorder at home. It reinforced the idea that if these were my last thoughts in life then, man, my life had been crap.

Another two hours later, after I had successfully completed my ceiling tile-counting task, the doctor came in to advise me that all my tests were clear. She admitted she'd never seen a healthier specimen of a man. (Clearly *she* had noticed the sit-ups.) 'Only,' she continued ominously, 'there seems to be a strange anomaly with your BSK counts.'

Okay, the doc may not have actually said 'BSK' — it could've been ING or AMP for all I knew. But whatever the BSK counts were, and no matter how high, low or unimpressive they managed to be, she didn't seem to be too concerned. And neither did I. In fact, I hadn't really been all that worried about my chest pains the entire time. I was only here because a woman (or three, in fact) had sent me to a doctor.

So, feeling awkward about occupying a bed that could better serve one of the screaming, bleeding patients still waiting for their diagnosis in the reception area, I suggested I leave. The doctor was hesitant at first but soon came around to my way of thinking. Her final words — and I remember them to this day — were as follows: 'Go home and get some rest. But if you do suddenly die of a heart attack in the middle of the night tonight, be sure to call us. I'd love to find out what was causing it.'

And with that kind message of love and support echoing in my mind, I made my way back into my pants and out of the emergency ward. It was 1am and I had to get home and out of those press-stud stickers before anyone saw me.

Today, I am proud to announce that I didn't die of a heart attack that night. My clock radio served as a morning wake-up call and I rolled out of bed to begin my new life. Which is exactly the same as my old one, but with fewer sit-ups. A man could have a heart attack doing that much exercise, you know.

# 3
# THE PSYCHOLOGIST

As a rule, depression is no laughing matter — the very notion of humour goes against every basic principle of such a condition. But sometimes the incompetence of others can be so amusing that it forces the sufferer to break through the darkness, highlighting, if only for a moment, that life isn't as bleak as you might imagine. Better still, if these incompetent folk are so ridiculously, comically hopeless that it makes you see life in a whole new light, they can almost cure you forever.

When I was twenty-six years of age, I suffered for around a year with clinical depression. A doctor prescribed me with an antidepressant to try to alleviate my malaise, while my girlfriend of the time, failing to realise the gravity of the situation, insisted that a dose of vitamins and some more exercise were all that was needed. After a few months with little to no change in my demeanour my lovely partner conceded that perhaps things were more serious than she had first anticipated. My problems were obviously beyond the healing capabilities of the Mega-Strength Multivitamins for Men she'd purchased for me, as good as they were.

To her credit, my girlfriend was an extremely intelligent woman. It was no real surprise to hear that she had already called a psychologist in my area and booked a time for me to visit him. The advantage of making the arrangements without my knowledge, she correctly anticipated, was that I would be far more likely to keep the appointment and get professional help than I would if she was just advising me to show up. No, this was set in stone now and I was too depressed and lethargic to cancel it. Plus, she had given the visit the added advantage of being on a weekday, meaning I would have to take time off work, something she knew I relished. And best of all, it was a Monday. Nobody wants to work on a Monday, depressed or otherwise.

I arrived in the psychologist's waiting room, dutifully on time, to be greeted by absolutely no one. As first impressions go, this did not instil much confidence. Leaving a depressed patient in an unstaffed waiting area was, as I saw it, a recipe for trouble. Take one young man lacking confidence and self-worth, mix with a touch of paranoia, stir for a few moments in a large, empty room, and watch as the condition rises.

After a minute or two of feeling as though I might not be worth greeting at the door, I sat down in a very uncomfortable chair and began flicking through what can only be described as the most useless range of magazines ever made available in a doctor's waiting room.

The mags in any doctor's lounge usually describes to me the person I'm about to meet. Doctors rarely go out to buy magazines for their clients, so I assume they merely bring in publications that they've purchased for themselves at some stage and no longer want. This guy had bought a copy of *Plant Life Magazine* sometime in 1984, apparently, and it continued to adorn his receptionist-less reception area years later when I stopped by. Perhaps it was cheaper than a real plant, which I noticed had escaped his purchasing abilities also.

Within a few minutes of me taking a seat, a man walked out of the bathroom. He had obviously been in there a while and looked relieved to have had some time alone. He was towelling his hands dry when he noticed me; he stepped forward and put out his moist palm to shake by way of introduction. Well, at least it was clean.

The man introduced himself as Manfred and seemed to have a fairly pleasant demeanour. He was slightly stocky, suggesting that he worked too many hours to bother with going to a gym, had grey hair and a set of comically thick glasses. Manfred immediately apologised for not having a receptionist there that day — she was on holiday in Fiji. Obviously the fees here weren't going to be cheap if clients were funding overseas holiday jaunts for the staff.

Manfred led me up a small flight of stairs without speaking a word, past two very large and well-decorated offices, and headed into what could easily have been mistaken for the broom cupboard. The only thing separating it from an actual broom cupboard seemed to be the lack of a broom. It was small, poorly lit, and had two chairs.

The walls were blank, save for a small poster that may or may not have been the centrefold in *Plant Life Magazine*. I normally look for some sort of framed qualification or diploma on the walls of my doctors' offices, but this guy had nothing. Surely this couldn't be good. I mean, even if he hadn't actually studied his profession, I would've been happy with a signed note from his mum — MANFRED IS VERY GOOD. JUST GIVE HIM A CHANCE. But there was nothing.

After a few moments spent gathering his things and his mind, Manfred finally spoke. He started by giving me his card and told me that I should hang on to it so I could book further appointments. This is never a good sign of a man's abilities. He was openly announcing that this visit would cure nothing, and that even he was aware that I'd have to come back and try again. To me, this is as stupid as telling a waiter the moment you arrive

THE PSYCHOLOGIST   **29**

in his restaurant that you won't be leaving a tip. Either way, you can be assured of crap service.

One thing I noticed on Manfred's decoration-free card was that it stated he specialised in 'teen counselling and marijuana addiction'. I don't know if this meant he was a specialist with teens because he was addicted to marijuana, or whether his office was simply a good place to score some gear. Either way, I feared I might be out of his league.

'So how old are you, Troy?' asked Manfred sincerely.

'I'm twenty-six,' I replied.

He looked confused already. I don't think my age should have been a surprise to him as I never glowed with any youthful exuberance and my manly, two-day facial growth clearly gave away the fact that I'd left high school a good many years earlier.

'And are you on any non-prescription medication ... if you know what I mean?' he continued.

'No.' Of course, I neglected to inform him of my Mega-Strength Multivitamins for Men and hoped he wouldn't notice my robust jittering.

'Ah ...'

Manfred seemed completely lost now and I immediately felt sorry for him. I wanted to clarify that I was suffering from depression, but something told me that it might be rude to assume he couldn't discover this for himself through his intense line of questioning. Then again, I wasn't paying this man to give me a diagnosis. I already had that. I was looking for a cure.

'Manfred, I've been told that I am suffering from severe biological depression,' I offered. 'I don't know where it stems from and I was hoping we could talk about causes and triggers for this kind of thing.'

Manfred now seemed more perplexed than ever. He may have been a little excited as well. Finally, a real patient!

'So, you don't take any drugs at all then?' he asked.

'No,' I repeated.

'Well, we need to look at what is causing your problem then.' At least he was speaking with some confidence now. 'When did this start?'

'Possibly about two years ago, but I only started having panic attacks about four months ago. My GP put me onto some antidepressant tablets to calm me down, but I still feel as though I have a problem.'

'And what would that problem be?'

'I'm depressed.'

'Ahh ...'

This line of questioning was going nowhere. Manfred had obviously never watched a decent spy thriller in his life. In a spy movie, anyone captured by this man would have no trouble keeping government secrets from him (unless, of course, they were a teenager with a drug habit).

Manfred was writing in a book as we spoke. I figured he must've put two large crosses next to his first two questions and was now desperately trying to fill in a blank page in order to look busy. Perhaps he had simply written: LOOK UP 'BIOLOGICAL DEPRESSION' BEFORE THIS GUY MAKES ANOTHER APPOINTMENT.

'So what do you do for a living, Troy?' he began again.

'I work for a marketing company,' I replied.

'And what's that like?'

'It's okay, I guess. It's not what I really want to be doing, but it pays the bills.'

'Well Troy, maybe you need to look at doing something that you truly enjoy. Something where money doesn't matter,' said Manfred, grasping at straws.

'But then how do I pay my bills?'

'Ahh ...'

I was getting used to the word 'ahh'. This man seemed to use it whenever he was stumped. He usually worked with teenagers,

I gathered, the majority of whom probably still lived at home. Issues like rent and paying for food were not high on their priorities, as they were provided free, no doubt. Not in my case, though.

'Well, you don't want to quit your job then,' continued Manfred, changing direction very quickly. 'Not until you've found another way to subsidise your lifestyle.'

'That's true.'

'So what else can you do?'

I thought about this for a while. Manfred seemed happy that a lot of the time was now being spent in silence. He didn't have to 'ahh' as much.

'Perhaps I could be a builder or something.'

'Do you like that kind of work?' he asked, desperately.

'No,' I replied.

'Ahh ...'

There it was again.

'Well, what do you enjoy?'

'I don't really know. That's my problem, I guess — nothing seems all that great right now. I don't feel as though I'm learning anything or experiencing life. I feel like I'm just an onlooker.'

I don't know what caused me to offer so much information all at once, nor why I'd made the mistake of using the word 'learning' in front of a counsellor for school-age individuals. Manfred's powers of interrogation hadn't warranted this kind of response, by any means, but his eyes lit up excitedly now. I knew where this was going.

'You say that you don't feel like you are learning anything,' he said. 'Perhaps you need to go back and study something.'

No, perhaps you should go back and study something! I desperately wanted to yell. But I didn't. That would've been cruel. He was only doing his job to the best of his abilities, as limited as they were.

'Maybe you should think about doing a course,' he continued, the glint in his eye becoming almost too bright to stare directly into.

Having announced this, Manfred also immediately announced that our time was up. As far as my interrogator was concerned, he had plumbed the depths of my soul, grabbed the problem by its ornate handles, and returned to the surface desperate for air but holding his prize aloft, like a diver who'd just found the treasures of Atlantis.

As he showed me to the door, Manfred advised me that he wanted me to do some homework before our next session. In my opinion, he made two major errors here. One, in thinking that any teenager with schooling issues and a marijuana addiction — or a 26-year-old with Mega-Strength Multivitamins for Men cravings — would ever want to indulge in any form of homework. And two, that there would even be a 'next session'.

He shook my hand again, that glint in his eye now able to light homes in times of a blackout, and bade me farewell. He reaffirmed that he had given me his card already, and led me out into the street, where I was finally alone again, no richer for the experience of having met him.

My girlfriend, in her genuine grief at her partner's mental regression, had sadly missed the mark on this one. I was grateful that she'd bothered to try, and Manfred, now $80 richer, was probably grateful to my girlfriend as well. I imagined him back inside the broom cupboard, flicking through a medical textbook, looking up 'biological depression' and realising by just how much he too had missed the mark.

I hurried onto the bus home, concerned that he might run out to me at any moment, eager to start the session again with his new-found knowledge. Or maybe just to sell me some ganja.

Lying on my floor at home, I couldn't help but laugh at the man's incompetence. Even when you're depressed, there's still something funny in the stupidity of others. As for an actual cure for my problems, I tried to think of a different angle. I needed something extreme. Something out of the ordinary that could change my way of thinking and shake my mind clear of this dark, depressing cloud that now came with a daily chance of mental thunderstorms.

Perhaps, I thought, I needed to be hypnotised.

# 4
# HYPNOTHERAPY
# PART I

Let me start by saying that the very next paragraph could very well shatter any illusions you may have about hypnotherapy. So if you wish to preserve your preconceived fantasies about such a profession, you might want to skip ahead. For those of you still here, my apologies for doing this, but it simply must be done.

There are no sequins.

There, I've said it.

In fact, not only are there no sequins, there was also no mustachioed man in a top hat dangling a large pocket watch in front of my eyes, saying, 'You are getting veeery sleepy ...'

Nothing!

The man about to conduct my less than magical hypnotherapy session was Dr Cho — a balding, portly man, wearing the most ludicrous pair of tiny glasses that looked as though they had been stolen from a plastic doll.

He was also a very repetitive man. He was a very repetitive man. He was a *very* rep—

I'm sorry, I got caught up in his vibe just then. But the honest truth is that Dr Cho told me the same, incomplete story no less than three times before beginning the therapy proper.

The scenario he described involved a man standing on the edge of a cliff — a nondescript character whom I gradually came to envisage as a balding, portly man with ludicrously tiny glasses and a memory problem. He then advised me that there were two possible opinions this man could have regarding his current situation, apparently: 'This outlook in front of me is fantastic' or 'This is too high — I could fall and lose my life.'

Dr Cho had neglected the possibility of a third option, namely, 'Damn, why did she throw my car keys all the way down there?' But I decided not to inform him of this, as he seemed to be struggling enough as it was.

After a completely unnecessary re-run of the cliff-top story, which was yet to have a conclusion of any sort, let alone a recognisable moral, Dr Cho chose to begin his version of depression therapy. I must admit, I was looking forward to this, and was disappointed that he wasn't wearing a cape or accompanied by a beautiful assistant named Sharon.

He was ruining my entire preconception of his art, in fact. As mentioned, there was no watch on a chain. There was no eerie music in the background. And, most tragically, there was no fantastical trigger word like 'Constantinople' to set off a series of hilarious events in the future.

Dr Cho's form of hypnotherapy merely required me to lie back in a well-worn reclining leather seat and become totally aware of the fact that I was breathing. I thought I'd always been aware that I was breathing — just not to the same level, say, as when an elderly relative is breathing loudly beside me while eating a sandwich. As it turned out, with the good doctor's coaxing, I was about to become this elderly relative, only without the food.

First he encouraged me to focus my awareness on one nostril. The left one, if I recall correctly. The tiny itching and tickling below my nostril indicated a waywardly long hair that urgently needed plucking. This was a medical office, surely there would be tweezers somewhere close by ...

Ignoring this minor distraction, I gradually became aware of a second nostril. Deep breaths were now flowing through both of my nasal blowholes, and slowly I began to drift away into a place of serenity and comfort. Dr Cho spoke quietly and with a monotonal slur, which encouraged this feeling of peace, as did the level of boredom on my part. He asked me to become aware of my leg muscles and to relax them thoroughly. Next, he described the tension in my arms and head, and then suggested I free them of any pressure or stress.

By the time he had explained to me the need to relax my buttocks, I was almost gone. Somewhat unnerved by the possibility that this level of relaxation could induce me to break wind, I was overcome with a strange feeling that the room I was in could've been anywhere on earth. The clock on the wall, which I had previously been deeply aware of, due to its loud ticking, seemed to tick no more. Perhaps the batteries had run out.

Darkness had descended upon me and my mind was drifting through other worlds. Beautiful colours adorned my dreams and half-dressed women danced provocatively as I floated above the clouds, then off through time and space. Just as one of the women reached over to me, urging me to release her from her restrictive clothing, I felt a sudden jolt on my shoulder.

My eyes flicked open and were filled with an offensive amount of light. Dr Cho stood over me — still clothed in whatever restrictive clothing he'd been wearing earlier, I was pleased to note. The latter allowed me a sigh of relief that I hadn't been acting out my recent fantasies.

'Are you okay?'

'I guess so,' I replied, a little startled. 'Did it work? Am I cured?'

'Well,' he began, amusement obvious in his face, 'you were completely relaxed. So relaxed that it seems you actually fell asleep before we could start the therapy.'

How embarrassing. I had used this man's office as a guest-house, reclining in his comfortable chair, imagining I was watching a dull show on TV, before drifting off to sleep. Chances are I broke wind at some stage too. The fact that he'd turned on his office fan seemed to indicate this might be true.

'I'm sorry,' I said, though not truly sure what I was sorry about. I mean, this short trip to the land of nod was setting me back close to $100 — I could've achieved that on my own for a fraction of the cost.

'It's okay. It happens to a lot of people the first time. What you have to become aware of is total relaxation while remaining awake. It isn't that hard.'

Sure, maybe not for him. He was a professional.

'Shall we try it again?' Dr Cho suggested.

'Okay, doc.' Hell, what other option did I have?

Dr Cho proceeded to relay the tediously familiar tale of the man on the cliff again, before lulling me back into a state of relaxation. This time I was fortunate enough to hear him count backwards from ten, presumably implying that by the time he said 'zero', I was completely under his power. It was like being anaesthetised, but without the cocky anaesthetist making you believe you'd never hear numbers seven through to one.

This time I managed to stay awake during the therapy exercise. But it didn't *feel* like I was awake. While there were no scantily clad women tempting me with their wares now, I was certainly not in my usual state of mind. It was calming, serene, and I could still hear the ticking on the wall. Surely that was a good sign.

Suddenly, within minutes of reaching this Eden, things started to go horribly wrong. Dr Cho was talking to me from what seemed like 4 miles away through a tin can connected to a piece of string. His voice was becoming too muffled to understand, and without any provocation from my thought patterns, everything started to rock violently. It was as if the comfortable leather recliner had mysteriously been transported to a rough part of the ocean and was being tossed around wildly while I held on for dear life.

Part of me realised that this wasn't how the therapy should be working; and, if it was, then it wasn't the kind of therapy I was after. Seasickness never cured anything except one's feeling of wellbeing, as far as I was aware.

But before I could make any adjustments to my psychic surroundings, the fully reclined seat of comfort sprung back from its position of rest and violently launched me forwards onto the floor in front of a startled Dr Cho.

'Are you all right?' he asked. 'The chair is getting old and it does that sometimes. I am sorry.'

Lucky I wasn't on the edge of that cliff he'd been banging on about ...

'I'm okay,' I replied, picking myself up from the floor. 'It wasn't so much the chair — it was the rocking backwards and forwards like I was on a boat that pissed me off. I couldn't make it stop.'

'You weren't moving at all, as far as I could see. Your mind may have made you *think* you were rocking, but you certainly weren't moving physically ... Hmm, that's not good.'

Not good? It was bloody awful. It made me feel nauseous. I'd say 'not good' was a massive understatement, buddy!

'Why is that not good?' I asked pathetically.

'Well, it does happen on rare occasions to people being hypnotised, but it sort of implies that you're not in a state of calm.'

I could've told him that, but instead I said, 'So what do we do now?' I was half expecting him to grab a straitjacket from the cupboard and tell me I was going to be taken off to a happier place by some men in white coats.

'Oh, nothing for now,' he replied lazily. 'We're out of time here today, but I really think you should come back next week and we can sort things out then.'

Hey, that's the reason I came here today, pal. What was this, a rehearsal? Is there a different fee structure for that? Will Sharon be here for the main show?

There were so many things I wanted to ask him, but the fact that he was already out of his chair and motioning towards the exit implied that my questions were no longer welcome. I was left to wonder what had been achieved exactly, other than a spectacular attempt to get me airborne from the comfort of a leather seat. If things didn't work out with his practice, the doctor and I could probably take our act on the road. I could just see 'Mysterious Cho and the Flying Troy Harvini' bringing joy and laughter to scores of small children across the land.

For no particular reason, I figured I'd give him one more chance before ordering the leotards and safety nets. If nothing else, I felt wonderfully rested, and for that he was still in my favour. Something told me this goodwill would not be lasting long, though.

# 5
# HYPNOTHERAPY
# PART II

The world's best hypnotism joke goes something like this:

First man: 'I went to my doctor to get hypnotised a couple of months ago.'

Second man: 'Really? Did it work?'

First man: 'No — and I tell him that every Wednesday when I go over to wash his car.'

I actually have a friend who wants to undergo hypnotism in order to help him quit smoking. But he's frightened that the practitioner will take advantage of him and leave him clucking like a chicken every time someone claps their hands. In my case, this was never a concern. Dr Cho simply wasn't that good.

Whatever it was that made me go and see him again is something I'll never understand. His attempt to hypnotise me a week earlier had been far from successful, but I had to keep trying to find a cure for my state of woe. I felt that something had to work eventually. Surely someone, somewhere, held the key to my happiness.

Could it be Dr Cho?

Having said that, curiosity played a big part in my decision as well. I'd always wondered what it would be like to be hypnotised. That, and Dr Cho's promise that he would teach me self-hypnosis soon, which I'd be able to use at any time. I had visions of being able to hypnotise away intense pain, should it ever befall me, or train my mind to believe I was twice as intelligent as I really was. At the very least, it might help me to enjoy broccoli. There had to be some use for it.

On arriving in his office, I sat down rather nervously in the weathered leather recliner. Dr Cho assured me that he'd taken a look at its spring mechanism and that last week's little 'event' would not occur again. Something in his voice made me doubt that he'd done anything more than stare down the back of the thing and give it a swift kick, before walking away defiantly as if he'd taught it a lesson.

Again Dr Cho began with the story of the man on the cliff. I started to wonder if this tale was simply designed to make my mind weary enough to manipulate. It was a dull story the first time I heard it, and it certainly wasn't getting any better with age.

By the time we got to the actual hypnosis side of things, I was practically asleep again. Depression had been keeping me up at night; I'd been worrying about what kind of permanent effect this ongoing sadness might have on me, so any opportunity to pass out under the watchful eye of a medical professional was extremely tempting. I managed to keep my eyelids from drifting down too heavily, however, and listened as Cho's monotonal voice counted back from ten to one, at which point I was apparently hypnotised.

It was odd, because I didn't feel any different compared to when I'd been sitting there, with my eyes lightly shut, becoming aware of my nostrils. I spent the next few moments in silence, trying to decide whether I had really gone under his spell or not. Perhaps I was dancing around his office making chicken noises — I'll never really know. But it certainly felt like I was still lying back in the dubious recliner, trying every trick in the book not to fart or drift into the land of slumber.

Dr Cho had obviously done this many times before, but I wondered if he'd ever had a patient suddenly throw their eyes wide open and yell '*Surprise!*' when he thought he had them under. I really wanted to do that. I believe I could have too, but perhaps that was part of the spell.

'So Troy, what you need to do is find a place,' he told me. 'A place in your mind where you are totally at home.'

'But not my home?' I asked, feigning drowsiness, as if to complete the ruse that he might actually have hypnotic ability.

'Ah … no. Not your *actual* home. Somewhere where you feel completely at ease. This place doesn't even have to exist — you can make it up from places you have seen or thought about. Make it the best possible place for you. When you have thought of this place, I want you to describe it to me.'

I paused for a while to gather my thoughts. Which was probably just as well, because my first impulse was to describe the Playboy Mansion, nude models and all. Hell, I think I'd feel at home there. Soon enough though, the surroundings and present company made me rethink my dream home and my mind began to wander.

What happened next is something I don't consider to be therapy. My mind wandered to my 'happy place'. I could visualise it completely, down to every last detail — and I didn't like what I saw. My imagination had conjured up a friend's holiday house on the beach: a palatial place so enormous and extravagant it made Trump Tower look like a tin shed. The floorboards were polished to an incredible shine, the balcony looked out over the water, giving a view of heavenly proportions, while girls in bikinis strolled by at regular intervals as if to advertise themselves as potential co-owners of this grand abode to the young, good-looking man of the house.

Having described this scene aloud in minute detail, I took a moment to reflect on what I'd envisaged. Sure, maybe it was the hypnotherapy leading me down some sort of path, but by this stage I was convinced that I was under no 'spell' as such. Rather, I was a man lying in a chair with his eyes closed, daydreaming.

'Stand on the balcony,' Dr Cho instructed.

'Sure. I'm there. I'm looking out at the water.'

'Now what are you thinking?' he asked vaguely.

'Um … nice water?'

'That's good, Troy. Very good. Are you frightened at all that you might fall off this balcony?'

Holy shit! Dr Cho had just attempted to make me the guy from his annoying cliff-top story, albeit in a different setting, one of my choosing. I hated that story with a passion by now, and I certainly didn't want to be in it.

I got what he was driving at, of course. We are all capable of making choices in our lives regarding our outlook; you can see the beauty or the fear in every situation, and it's up to you to decide. But it didn't require two sessions of supposed hypnotherapy to drill that into me — the point was clear enough the very first time he'd told me the story.

Worse still, he had made me realise that my happy place was, in fact, someone else's property. Somewhere that I would never own. If I was depressed before, this little nugget of information was only going to compound the problem.

'You can start to relax again and come back to the real world as I count back from ten, okay Troy?' the doc threw in.

'No,' I replied stubbornly. I wasn't hypnotised, I wasn't being led in any way by his gentle suggestions, and I certainly wasn't cured, by any stretch of his limited imagination. So I decided to have some fun.

'What do you mean, *no?*' asked Dr Cho, nervously.

'I'm staying here. I like the view too much.'

'Oh ... Well, perhaps we can go back there next time you're here.'

I felt bad at this point, I admit. Dr Cho was trying to help me and no doubt genuinely believed he had the ability to hypnotise people. Who was I to come in and shatter that illusion?

'Okay,' I said, opening my eyes before he could talk me through the recovery process.

He looked a little stunned. 'You okay?' he asked.

'Yeah, doc. I'm fine.'

And I was fine. Not great, not outstanding, not wholly satisfied with life — but perfectly fine, nonetheless.

This man's inability to hypnotise me, twice, combined with Manfred the psychologist's failure to do anything at all with any level of competence had taught me that even the most qualified professionals are merely winging it in life.

And the sudden realisation that this lesson brought me eased my mind about my own existence. Perhaps I hadn't discovered my place on the planet quite yet, but part of me felt a lot better knowing that those who apparently had were simply making it up as they went along.

There was a great comfort in that. Two men of limited ability had inadvertently set me on the path to recovery from depression. One of them had also launched me across the room like a circus performer.

Looking back, I'm surprised more wasn't said of that event. Was it part of the therapy? Had Dr Cho planned the human-cannonball episode from the start?

I'd like to think he had. The very notion that one of his supposed cures might've been to just belt a patient hard like a faulty electronic device reinforces the idea that he really wasn't sure what he was doing. But, like everyone else, he had to try, didn't he?

Because, who knows, something might actually go right once in a while.

# 6
# STILL SWEATY AFTER ALL THESE YEARS

I am one sweaty sonofabitch. I sweat for absolutely no reason. I can be sitting, motionless at my office desk, under an ice-cool air-conditioning vent in summer or with a pleasant ocean breeze drifting in from my open window during winter, and still I'll be sweating — like the polar ice caps thanks to global warming.

Sweating, for me, is involuntary. Not that anyone volunteers to sweat, but generally you know when and why it's going to start. Either you're exerting yourself in the gym, or you're running for a bus, or you're on a first date and nervous as all hell because you stupidly ate bran muffins all afternoon and now you can suddenly feel things starting to shift. Whatever the reason, it's usually self-induced and you wear the appropriate clothing. For me, sweating occurs whenever it wants to. It doesn't matter what I'm wearing or who I'm trying to impress — my sweat does not discriminate.

This all began sometime in my teens. I was a pretty fit young man back then, a member of the local Surf Life Saving Club and also fairly active in occasional sports, so sweat wasn't a foreign concept to me. But over a period of a few months, I started to notice moisture under my arms and down my back more often when I wasn't actually partaking in any physical activity. One day, I guess, it just *began*.

Following this slow discovery and the immediate assumption that I was dying of something drastic, my friends teased me mercilessly about my supposed lack of fitness. Surely, they believed, if I was sweating profusely while sitting in the pub or walking between nightclubs, it was because I was a fat, lazy bastard with a penchant for slacking off. It made sense to them.

It didn't make sense to me, though. Not only was I as fit as I had ever been, I never felt exerted or exhausted when these sweat attacks came on. But try explaining that to a bunch of mates with bellies half-full of booze.

Eventually I accepted my fate. I came to the conclusion that my insides weren't overheating and boiling up due to some weird, alien disease, and simply went about my every day — constantly excusing myself whenever I left a sudden puddle on people's veranda. (That's no joke, by the way; it happened twice.)

But acceptance was one thing — it was still frustrating as hell, and remains so all these years later. Sweating tends to strike you when you want it to strike least. It leaks through your clothes and makes it incredibly difficult to keep your white shirts white. Oh, and worst of all, it makes women run for the hills.

Compounding the problem for me during my teenage years, this all came about before the internet had been fully embraced around the globe. Lest we forget, back in the early '90s, the world's information was not necessarily a keystroke away. It was hidden in libraries. So I couldn't simply type in my symptoms, press Search and discover that my affliction was actually quite a common one. That it was something I didn't have to be completely ashamed of and, potentially, something that could maybe one day be repaired. No, I could only find this out by visiting a ... [insert dramatic music] ... *doctor*.

As usual, my mother was the first one to suggest a trip to the local GP. She had heard me whine about being sweaty one too many times and was no doubt sick of my questions regarding the washing and soaking of badly stained white shirts. Mum passed me a card she'd obtained from a friend. It was the business card of a GP in the city who apparently dealt with 'weird problems'.

'He's very good,' she began. 'He cured Andy of something weird he had a few years ago that no one else could even understand.'

'Who's Andy?' I asked, instantly putting on my anti-doctor face.

'Andy! He's Madge's son.'

'Who's Madge?'

'She's your second aunty, twice removed on your father's side,' Mum explained, as though it was something I should've known. 'The point is, he's very good apparently and he might be able to help you with your sweating.'

She seemed to be slightly irked by my stubbornness, but there was something else I noticed. Mum had begun her approach by assuring me that this doctor was 'very good', only to then soften it with the word 'apparently' — the reason being, I was sure, that she'd be able to absolve herself of any responsibility should things go horribly wrong. My mum is a genius. I still have a lot to learn from this woman.

The doctor's name was Dr L Perensky, the 'L' remaining a mystery for the duration of our encounter. I made an appointment with his receptionist a mere week in advance and was alarmed at his availability at such short notice. If this guy was so brilliant at his job, then why didn't I have to book a year ahead? There should've been queues of people lining the streets, surely, begging for a moment with the great and mysterious L. Not only that, but he should've been located at the end of a yellow brick road, not in the basement of an 1850s building desperately in need of renovation.

I arrived at Dr Perensky's office a little alarmed at the lack of décor and care afforded his waiting room. It was stark and unwelcoming, with a clutter of old magazines scattered carelessly over a low, oval table and onto the floor. A fluorescent light flickered annoyingly overhead and the receptionist was nowhere to be seen.

I paused for a moment at the reception desk, half expecting someone to appear as a result of my deliberately loud shuffling. Nothing. So I moved over to one of the aged brown couches and noisily flicked through an ancient, crusty-paged gossip magazine. The cover actually featured the cast of *Charlie's Angels*. No, not the movie cast, the TV ones. From the 1970s. Brilliant.

A few articles into this printed time capsule, I was interrupted by the receptionist, who had made her way back to her post undetected, sitting herself down and trying to look as if she'd been there all along. The joke was on her, however, as I had sweated all over that desk a few minutes before. She seemed frustrated by the mysterious droplets, I noticed.

'Excuse me, have you checked in?' she enquired abruptly.

I assumed this woman was the only person on checking-in duties, so there was a very good chance she already knew what my reply would be. Regardless, I played along. 'Uh, no,' I said. 'There was no one here.'

'Are you Troy Harvey?'

'Yes.'

'Fine,' came the response. 'Dr Perensky will be with you in a minute.' She then promptly left the room again. Judging by the hurry in which she gathered her coat and handbag, it was hard to tell if she was simply leaving for lunch or had resigned for good.

I settled back into the couch I was slowly seeping through and flicked over a few more pages of my ancient magazine. There was an article about *Young Talent Time*. I kid you not.

Before long, a short man in his mid fifties entered the room, burping. He curled his hand into a fist and put it up to his chest. 'Excuse me,' he offered, 'I'm having some terrible reflux. *Beeerrp* ... Sorry. I'm Dr Perensky. Please, come into my office.'

What an introduction. I instantly started to wonder how good this doctor could be at curing the rare and incurable if he couldn't grasp the simplicity of reflux.

'Troy, what can I do for you?' he asked. '*Beeeerp* ... Sorry.'

'I've got a sweat problem,' I said matter-of-factly, pointing at my lubricated forehead.

'I see. Did you jog here or were you running late at all?' No burps this time. A good sign.

'No, in fact I came by taxi and I've been sitting in your waiting room. So nothing out of the ordinary. This happens all the time, actually — even when I'm not doing anything.'

'Yeah, I've seen this before. *Beeeeerrrrp* ... Whoa! Excuse me ... Have you ever had reflux? Terrible, terrible thing.'

'Um, no,' I replied unsympathetically. I wasn't here to talk about *his* problems.

'Right, right. Let me — *beeeerp* ... take a look in here ...' He then flicked through the pages of a large book, pausing briefly at the index and burping lightly into it, before flicking some more and alighting at the diagnosis he was looking for. 'A-ha! Now tell me, Troy, do you find yourself sweating from the palms of your hands at all?'

Sweaty palms? Ewwww.

'No. Not at all. Just my underarms, my back and my forehead. The normal sweat places,' I concluded, desperately hoping he would agree with my self-prognosis of normalcy.

'I see. And do you find you *beerrrrrp* ... oh ... sweat more if you're stressed or nervous about something?'

'I've never noticed. I mean, I get stressed when it starts and sometimes I think that makes it worse, but I don't really know. I'm just sick of it and was wondering how I could stop it.' To tell the truth, I was hoping for a tablet or an elixir of some nature that would resolve this problem once and for all.

'You have a condition called hyperhidrosis,' he declared.

'I see,' I said, not seeing at all.

'Basically, it's exactly as it sounds — *hyper*, meaning overactive, and *hidrosis*, meaning hydration or liquid.'

That didn't help me at all. 'Yes, I already know I sweat hyperactively — but how can I stop it?'

'Well ... *beeeerrrrp* ... you can't, I'm sorry. I mean, it's not something that is very easy to control.'

'What do you mean, not *easy* to control? You *can* control it, can't you?' I was starting to get very nervous now.

'Uh ... *beeerrrrp* ... no. Not really. There is one way, but it involves a very delicate operation and the severing of the nerves in your spine.'

Severing my spine? Hmmmm, let me think about that for a moment ...

'Nope!' I replied hastily. 'No spine severing, thanks.'

'Good choice.' He was half laughing as he said it. 'It's not the most successful operation on record. A lot of patients have had complaints afterwards.'

'You mean like being unable to walk and stuff?' I asked, a touch sarcastically.

'Not exactly. But think of it like this. Your body has over-productive sweat glands. Basically, the sweat glands are designed to cool down the body whenever it overheats. What happens is, a signal is sent via the nerve ending to the glands to produce the sweat and cool the body — simple. The problem is, though, once we sever the nerves, they no longer send the signal to the sweat glands in your underarms and on your forehead, so where does the signal go?'

I wasn't sure if he wanted me to answer the question or not. He left such a long gap. 'Um ... your brain?' I said eventually.

'No. They *come* from your brain, Troy ... No, the body still needs to cool down, so it simply resends the signal somewhere else after it gets no response from the usual outlets.'

'Like where?' I was actually becoming quite interested now that he'd stopped with the belching.

'Well, we had one guy complain that the sweat was now pouring out of his thighs and crotch. On his wedding day he experienced excessive sweating and spent the entire wedding in wet pants, much to the amusement of his mates.'

Holy shit! 'So what did he do?' I asked, feeling terrible for the poor sweaty-pants guy. 'Can you fix it?'

'I'm afraid not. Once you sever a nerve in your spine, it can't be undone. I hear they're working on a reversible method where they simply clamp the nerve, but no one's perfected it yet. Anyway, it's too late for that guy,' he ended, smiling.

How could he smile at such a situation? That poor guy would be walking around in wet pants for the rest of his life, desperately trying to explain to anyone and everyone that he hadn't in fact pissed himself. I'll bet his marriage didn't last too long either.

'Well, if I'm going to sweat,' I responded, 'I'd rather sweat from the more acceptable sweaty outlets. You know — the ones where people instantly know it's only sweat.'

'I agree!' At this, Dr Perensky leapt up from his seat excitedly and returned the large book to its shelf.

'So that's it? There's nothing I can do?'

'Well, pretty much, I'm sorry to say. You can try using deodorants with a high aluminium content. That helps in some cases.'

'Yeah, but I can't exactly spray that on my forehead, can I?'

'Oh ... I never thought of that. I suppose not.'

There was an awkward pause.

'So ... is that it?' I asked again, desperately hoping he was withholding the magical elixir.

'I'm afraid so. But, at least you know what it is now. That's something, right?'

'Sure.' In fact, all I could be sure about was that I was destined to be a sweaty mess for the rest of my days.

I stood up and made my way back out to the depressing waiting room, where a new, just-as-bored receptionist was filing her nails at the reception desk. Looking over my shoulder, I half thanked Dr Perensky as he shuffled back into his office, smiling and waving and no doubt soon to enjoy another bite of whatever sandwich had earlier ravaged his oesophagus.

The receptionist barely looked up as she took my payment and asked under her breath if I needed to make another appointment.

'What for?' I shot back despondently, before heading outside to leak some more onto the world.

Years on from that appointment with the burping Dr L Perensky, I'm still a sweaty mess. Not always, but often enough for it to get on my nerves. One such occasion was when I was acting in a cheap TV commercial under extremely hot lights. Any normal person would've started to perspire after a little while. Me, I saw the lights from my dressing room and proceeded to lubricate the entire set before I'd even arrived on it, letting go a tidal wave of underarm secretion that could have destroyed the electrical equipment. The shoot eventually had to break every eight minutes and put me in front of a fan to cool down for fifteen minutes before going back out for another eight. By the end, a standard four-hour shoot had taken nine hours to complete. No one was impressed, least of all me.

By the way, they have managed to perfect the spine-clamping operation since then, although I'm still too chicken to give it a try. Aside from the horror of having a clamp put on your spine, the mere thought of sweaty testicles twenty-four hours a day is enough to stop any man from undergoing such an ordeal, I'd say.

All up, hyperhidrosis is not really as bad as it sounds. It's just a bit of sweat every now and then. And while that puts some people off occasionally, at least people aren't walking around thinking I've pissed myself.

# 7
# THE GUY ACTUALLY CUT ME

It was sometime around Christmas several years ago when I found myself lying shirtless next to my girlfriend, dozing in the warm, early hours of the morning. At some stage during my slumber, I must've rolled over onto my stomach, revealing my bare back to my girlfriend.

'You have a red lump on your back,' she announced far too loudly for that time of day.

Why she was even looking at my back while I slept, I don't know, but at that hour I didn't particularly care what she did. 'Mmmph,' came my pathetic reply.

'Can I squeeze it?' she begged.

'Mmmph.'

I was pretty sure that noise meant 'no', but instead she took it as an open invitation and pounced on my back like a professional hunting-lobster. Then she began to squeeze my skin furiously, digging her pincers into me and thoroughly waking me from my blissful half-sleep.

'Go easy!' I cried, struck by sudden pain.

'I'm trying, but it seems a bit deep. I really want to get it.'

'And I really want to walk again!' I replied. 'I think you might be squeezing out my spine, you know.' It really did hurt. I'm not normally that pathetic.

'No, no — it's coming!' She squealed with delight.

Then, suddenly — *pow!* The contents shot out and hit her on the forehead. (Yes, you read that correctly.)

Believe it or not, my girlfriend actually thought this entire event was amazing. 'This is amazing!' she yelled.

Now, those aren't the words you'd normally expect to hear from your partner in this situation. On previous occasions when a girlfriend of mine had been kind enough to squeeze a nasty pimple on my back, the adjective accompanying 'This is' tended to be one or more of the following: disgusting, gigantic, foul, gross, like Vesuvius, revolting, or even 'in the exact shape of Mary MacKillop', but never 'amazing!'

'You should see this, Troy. It's still coming! It never stops!'

She was more excited than I'd ever seen her. I could've saved a fortune in trying to impress her with jewellery in the past if I'd known I had this gift on my lower back.

'Wow!' she went on as the fluids continued to fly.

And continue they did for thirty-seven continuous minutes. That's more than half an hour of non-stop pus, like a radio station pumping out all the zits, commercial-free. That really *is* amazing. And disgusting.

Finally, the well of pus dried up, the show was over, and there lay my little princess thoroughly exhausted. I was in agony and she was sweating like she'd just given birth. 'What *was* that?' she asked, assuming I'd been keeping it a secret.

'How should I know? I've never even seen it.'

'Hmm. Perhaps you should go and see a doctor about that.'

I let out an audible sigh but knew it would do absolutely no good. I was powerless against those magic words.

Straight away, I got off the bed, threw on some clothes and headed up to the local medical centre, where I was unceremoniously partnered with a humourless doctor of considerable age. In fact, he may have been the walking dead with some sort of grudge against the living. That grudge, it would turn out, involved me and my fun-filled back.

After explaining to Dr Wise the gruesome details of my recent eruption, he stared at me blankly. The guy didn't even flinch. I was doing somersaults on the floor, acting out the story for him and ... nothing. At one stage I played the part of the pus, launching myself across the room for his benefit, but still no response. It was only after my one-man show was over that he leaned forward in his chair to address me.

'You have a cyst,' he said calmly.

'Okay ... Er, what does that mean, exactly?'

Dr Wise let out a deep huff as if to let me know that describing the problem wasn't actually part of his job and I probably should've arrived better prepared. Luckily, he continued. 'It's a big one. It probably began as a pore that got blocked and has since become infected. It will have to be removed so we can see if it's dangerous.'

How could a pus-filled sac be dangerous? I wondered. So far, it had only attacked my girlfriend out of self-defence. I doubted it would take control of my brain and force me to do things against my will, like rob a bank or release country-music albums. How could it be dangerous to others? Of course, that's when the realisation hit me: it could be dangerous to *me*.

Now, I don't consider myself a selfish man. Heck, part of the reason I don't like going to doctors is to spare them the hassle of having to deal with the likes of me. I try to do my best by others. But when something could actually affect my life — the one thing I can't really do without — well, frankly I become concerned.

THE GUY ACTUALLY CUT ME     57

I put on a brave face for the doctor. 'Will I have to go to hospital?' I was practically weeping.

'No, no,' he responded quickly. 'I'll do it here. Now.'

'Oh ... sure.'

'Follow me down the hall and take your shirt off,' he instructed, military fashion.

'Can I wait until we get there before I take my shirt off?' It was quite a long hallway and we'd be passing several other rooms to get to where we were going.

'Of course! Don't take it off *here*!' he replied, alarmed. And with that, Dr Wise set off down the hall at a cracking pace.

I broke into a light jog to keep up. 'So will this hurt?' I gasped, making good time.

'Not really.'

What did that mean exactly? Would there be a mythical hurt — a pain that could only be described in a Harry Potter novel? I mean, what the hell was 'Not really'?

After a short jog, we reached a room that looked identical to the one we'd just come from. The doctor again ordered me to de-shirt, adding, 'Place it on the chair and lie face down on the bench.'

I did so immediately, much to his disappointment.

'Wait a minute!' he hollered. 'I still have to put a sheet on the bench!'

I leapt up and stood in the corner while Dr Wise busied himself constructing this makeshift operating table. Judging by his military precision and tone, I expected it to have perfectly folded corners and no loose ends; but instead he simply shook out the white sheet and thrust it over the bench like a tablecloth, before motioning me to lie down again. It hardly seemed professional.

'First I'll give you a local anaesthetic to numb the area,' he informed me.

I have to say, it's usually at about this point that my nervous babbling with medical professionals really kicks in. I am terrified of being cut up or manipulated by doctors and instantly attempt to keep these situations as light and upbeat as possible.

'Local?' I asked, setting myself up for comedy gold. 'I'd actually prefer something more *international* if you've got it. I have expensive tastes.' Genius. Ladies and gentlemen, I'll be here all week. Please, tip your waitress!

'What?' the doctor asked gruffly.

'Uh, nothing. I ju—'

'Lie still.'

So there I lay, nervously staring into my pillow as another humourless doctor began working his magic on another part of my mysterious body. The local anaesthetic wasn't too painful and before long I could sense that, although I was without feeling, he was well into the task at hand. Again my nervousness kicked in.

'Do you need a hand back there, doc?' I offered, jokingly.

'Lie still!' This guy was offering nothing.

'Is it bad?' I tried again, eager to drown out the squelching noise that his surgical instrument was making.

No reply from the old man, only a question of his own: 'Can you feel anything?'

Either he was concerned that the anaesthetic might've worn off, or perhaps he was keen to pour some directly into my mouth.

'Nothing!' I replied honestly. 'In fact, I'd be surprised if you were doing anything at all back there. You're not just pretending to perform surgery so you can charge me a fortune, are you?'

Bad move. It was clearly a joke, as there were no charges for the work Dr Wise was doing right now. Everything was covered by some sort of medical insurance, so it made no difference to me financially if he was carving me up or not. And as it turned out, he was.

'Does it *look* like I'm just *pretending*?' he thundered, bringing his blood-soaked gloves to within an inch of my face.

I felt a wave of nausea, which instantly shut me up before I could utter another word.

'Good,' he said, shaking his head and returning to the site of the massacre.

What possesses me to blurt out such stupid things to medical professionals? Having said that, I still have to believe there are some doctors out there with a sense of humour. I've watched *Patch Adams*. I know they exist somewhere.

After seeing the mess on his surgical gloves, I decided it would be best if I buried my face in the pillow and attempted to smother myself, in the hope that I might black out until this frightful ordeal was over. But too soon, the old man interrupted my asphyxiation task with an alarming nugget of conversation.

'About the size of two golf balls,' he muttered to no one in particular.

'What?'

'The cyst. It's about the size of two golf balls. I've never seen one that big before.' He seemed impressed. 'Here ...'

At that point, a glass jar full of clear liquid appeared in front of my face. It contained the most disgusting, alien-looking creature I have ever laid eyes on. 'What the *fuck* is that?' I screamed, rolling backwards.

'That's your cyst,' he told me, grabbing my shoulder to roll my body forwards again. 'Don't roll backwards — I haven't stitched you up yet!'

Judging by the size of the creature in that jar, there must've been a pretty big hole in my back right now. I turned my head the other way to notice a mark of blood that had sprayed onto the wall. Feeling nauseous once more, I lay still as I was sewn back together like a damaged child's toy and listened as Dr Wise explained the next step.

'I'll send this down to pathology to make sure there's nothing weird about it, and you can call for the results in a few days, okay?'

Nothing weird about it, he says ... Apart from its giant, freaky appearance, I guess, and the fact that it was growing in a part of my body that doesn't normally harvest such hideous-looking creatures. *No, nothing weird at all.*

And this 'down to pathology' business — why are pathology labs always 'down'? We were currently in a ground-floor room and, as far as I knew, there was only a car park below us. So where are these elusive pathology workers — at the centre of the earth or something? Was Jules Verne merely a medical courier transporting body parts to the rarely seen mole-people of Pathology City? It intrigued me. Not enough to talk to this guy about it, mind you.

'What about the stitches?' I asked.

'Come back in a week and I'll take them out. You should be fine.'

'Great. Will it be painful when the anaesthetic wears off?'

'No. It should be fine,' he said again, as if to imply that any pain I might feel would merely be a result of my being a big girly-man.

I threw my shirt on, thanked him and left the room wondering more about the world than I had before I'd walked in. Everything seemed different. For one, I felt slightly lighter — two golf balls lighter, to be exact. I assumed this was how eunuchs felt.

My euphoria and wonder wore off approximately two hours later, at about the same time as the anaesthetic. This wasn't pain, this was *agony*. It was the kind of pain you get after having a limb severed by a searing-hot chainsaw (I imagine).

I lay face down on the bed, begging for my girlfriend to do something, anything, to put me in a state of unconsciousness.

'It'll be okay, baby,' she said in her adorable fashion. 'Hey, if you have to lie face down, do you want to me to check your back for pimples?'

'No!' I yelled, pulling my shirt down to prevent her evil hands gaining access to my flesh once again. She was the one who had started all this in the first place.

'Oh, you're being silly! How bad can it be?'

If only she knew.

If there can be an upside to this episode, it was that the fantastical underground pathology people found nothing 'weird' about my mutant back-baby and I was given the all-clear by my angry doctor a little less than a week later.

To this day I still have a super-cool scar down the middle of my back. If anyone asks, I tell them I was stabbed in a nightclub brawl in Kings Cross when I was a wild, reckless teenager. At least in that version of events I got to cut the other guy too.

# 8
# PINS AND NEEDLES

I hate that song that goes 'Feeling hot, hot, hot!' followed by a blast of flamboyant trumpets and loud, synthetic drums. I *always* feel hot and I don't need a song to remind me.

As previously explained, I sweat a lot. Now, if the body produces excessive amounts of sweat, that sweat needs to escape the body in order to prevent some sort of internal flooding, or something like that. As I learned from Dr Perensky years before, this is basically a cooling method for the body's core temperature, preventing it from reaching the same heat levels as the sun and, possibly, spontaneously combusting.

According to Dr Perensky, many patients who underwent spinal surgery initially celebrated the joy of no longer sweating excessively from their face and underarms and went about their daily lives with renewed confidence. *Initially*. For, as we saw in *Jurassic Park 2*, 'nature finds a way'. With the sweat unable to pour endlessly from their faces and pits, due to nerve laceration, it instead began making its way out of pores in their legs and their groins. Excessively so. Hence, the spinal-surgery option continued to hold no appeal for me. I mean, if I'm going to be drenched through perspiration, I'd like it to be in places where people instantly know it's sweat and nothing else.

This sweaty story, having begun during my teens, now resumes in my twenty-eighth year. It was sometime in the middle of one of those three endless summer months that my body despises more than others, and I was pouring with sweat even more than usual. It's generally out of my control from December to January, and frustrating in every way.

I was visiting my parents' house for lunch on a lazy Sunday afternoon and had been unable to refrain from cursing loudly when their ceiling fan groaned and grunted to a halt, leaving us all to endure the searing heat that God had provided that day, without relief. Seeing my dismay and hearing curse words that they'd long believed I never uttered, my mother enquired what solutions might be available for someone with my rapid-moistening ailment.

'Well, they can sever my spine,' I explained sarcastically.

She didn't like that one bit. 'Oh now, come on! How would you walk? That's madness.

'Well, that's the only solution,' I moaned. 'Some genius doctor you once sent me to told me so.'

'That seems a bit extreme,' Mum replied. 'What about seeing a naturopath? Your grandfather went to one and it helped him with a weird thing that his arm was doing.'

Great — so it seemed weird ailments ran in the family. Shouldn't someone have been studying our mutant genes by now, to prevent us from spreading these horrors to future generations?

'What the hell is a naturopath?' I asked. 'Sounds like a hippy doctor.'

'No, they're really good! I've seen one and he helped with a knee problem I was having. There's one just down the road here — I'll get you his card.'

Mum trundled off as I pondered what her knee trouble could possibly be, and why everyone in the family appeared to have medical issues that were incurable using modern medicine. What age were we living in?

I shot a desperate glance at my father. 'Don't look at me,' he said, shrugging his shoulders the way every man does once a woman suggests visiting a medical practitioner.

Turning back to see how my mum was doing with that card, I was instantly greeted by her hand in my face, holding the contact information of one Dr Nespith. For a woman with a troubled knee, she certainly moved swiftly.

'Call him on Monday,' she said forcefully. 'He's wonderful. He does everything, even acupuncture.'

I had never mentioned a desire to experience acupuncture in the past, so why was it suddenly brought up here? Was she hoping to heighten my curiosity about this man's healing powers or simply implying that he truly did have some kind of legitimate qualifications?

'So he's not just some weird hippy who makes you drink a freaky blend of tea so you can see into your own soul and find the cure within, is he?' I asked, making my dad laugh.

'Stop it!' yelled my mother. 'He's not a hippy. He's a *doctor*!'

Dad had gotten a taste now and was enjoying the mood. 'A witch doctor?' he said, conjuring another reaction from my mum.

'I give up ...' my mother sighed.

And so the family sat there exchanging the usual barbs and conversation until the day had passed and I headed home. The odd thing is, something stuck with me from that discussion. Mum's comment 'He does everything, even acupuncture' had tunnelled its way into my brain. I'm sure she said it for that very reason, because suddenly my mind was open to the idea of acupuncture as a possible cure for my excessive sweating. Since nothing else had worked, perhaps this was the miracle I'd been looking for in my leaky life. Hey, stranger things have happened.

First thing Monday morning, I phoned Dr Nespith's office and made an appointment for the following weekend. At first I was a little concerned, as I often am, that the abundance of available appointment times might've indicated few repeat customers — but maybe that was because he had cured them with one prick of his magic needles. Maybe? Possibly?

The week went by as weeks are duly appointed to do and in no time at all I found myself sitting in a strange man's lounge room, which was littered with pamphlets for rare herbs and alternative spiritual retreats. Dr Nespith's 'practice' turned out, in fact, to be nothing more than a three-bedroom home, using one of the bedrooms as an office and his actual lounge as a waiting area. There was no receptionist, no water cooler and not a dying plant to be seen. It was simply this man's house and, frankly, it made me uneasy.

I flicked through a few of the pamphlets scattered before me and wondered whether he put up with these brochures being strewn everywhere when he was chilling out in front of the TV after work. This was not a relaxing room for living in, yet not a proper waiting room either; it had no real feeling other than one of awkwardness. I could never sit back and watch *The Simpsons* here, for instance. (Mind you, on reflection, I could enjoy *The Simpsons* anywhere — so I take that back.)

Soon I was greeted by Dr Nespith and ushered into his so-called office. It was incredibly large for a spare room and the high ceilings gave it a rather grand appearance.

'Allo, Misser Harvey, how are you, sir?' he asked in an unidentifiable, yet thoroughly delightful accent.

'Actually, I'm fine,' I answered, surprised to hear myself make such a claim. 'Actually, that's not entirely true. I have a sweat problem. I sweat for no reason sometimes and can't make it stop.'

'Ziss is not a problem,' he replied, with a confidence I liked. 'Pleaze be giving me your hand, Misser Harvey.'

With his charming accent, how could I refuse?

'Ahhh, yez,' he said to himself, while violently rubbing the skin between my index finger and thumb.

'Ow,' I said casually, merely keen for something to say in such an awkward situation.

'Iz ziss hurting?'

'Um, no.'

'Zen why did you go "Ow"?'

'Um ... I don't know,' I said apologetically.

He sighed and continued to massage my hand. 'I am zeeing now the problem. It iz quite clear. What iz appening ere iz zat your liver and your lungz are zimply not communicating.'

I was stunned. 'Well, there's been a rift there for years!' I announced like a fool. 'In fact, the kidneys tried to get involved at one stage, to host an intervention, but it was no good. So if you can get them talking, then you're a better man than me!'

As the words were coming out of my mouth, I felt like the biggest dickhead in the world. I wasn't intentionally mocking this man and his ridiculous profession, but it was very hard for me to contain myself when presented with such hokum. Dr Nespith was not amused.

'Ahhh, am not following,' he said.

'Nothing ... It was nothing. I was just mucking around. Sorry.'

'It iz all right. I am telling you what iz the problem, that iz all.'

I felt now might be a good time to change the topic. 'So, that's quite an accent, doctor. Where are you from?'

Smooth move.

'I am from Iran,' he replied, offering little more than a disappointed glance in my direction as he opened a toolkit full to the brim with giant needles and other terrifying equipment.

Fuck.

Now, I'm not a racist man. I think racism is one of the most evil things to invade the minds of people on this planet, and I'm truly astonished when I hear people make statements about individuals based solely on their race. However, when a slightly agitated Iranian man opens up a toolkit of torture implements in front of you, given the way the world is behaving at present, it's hard for your mind not to drift over to the dark side of humanity, if only for a moment ...

Up until this point, Dr Nespith had been nothing but charming and warm, so I instantly dismissed these horrible thoughts from my mind. The strange thought that crept in now, though, was that I had never heard of an Iranian naturopath-cum-acupuncturist. I was sure they existed and I was sure they were extremely good at their jobs — it had just never crossed my mind before. That's all I'm saying.

He motioned for me to get up from my chair and move to the surgical bed in the middle of the room. 'Take off your shoez and shirtz and lie down,' he commanded, and I did. 'Now, pleaze roll up your zleeves and try to relax for me.'

*Relax.* The favourite word of doctors the world over. Man, if I'd been able to relax I wouldn't have been in a room with a medical person in the first place. And when a man I'd just made fun of had a bagful of needles he wanted to drive into me, I was going to be as far from relaxed as is humanly possible — trust me.

'I'll try,' I said with a smile, desperately attempting to rebuild the bridge of friendship.

'Ziss may hurt,' he warned, his tone implying that the bridge was still very much out.

*Needle one.*

'Ow!' I yelled.

Dr Nespith had placed the first needle in the gap between my big and second toe.

'I told you ziss may hurt. It will be okay. Yust relax.'

*Needle two.*

'Jesus!'

And so it continued, with excruciating pain each time, until my feet and arms were almost completely covered in needles. I looked like a half-man, half-metallic porcupine from a B-grade sci-fi movie. *Mancubine — defender of the forest!*

'Zere are yust a few more to go,' he said, turning off the lights.

Oh, you're kidding me — now the lights are off! Whatever happened to 'yust relax'? Here I was, completely at the mercy of a man I had possibly offended, covered in needles and in almost total darkness. I mean, at the very least, wouldn't he need the light to find the exact location for his next needle wound?

'Ow!' Apparently not.

This last needle had been inserted directly into the top of my skull. I shit you not. Right where the small bald patch appears in my increasingly unfashionable hairstyle.

'It iz okay. Ziss iz the one which is conducting all ze otherz,' Dr Nespith explained.

'Oh,' I replied, with zero understanding of what he was talking about.

'Yust relax ...'

Then, having finished, he made his way out of the room, closing the door behind him. He simply vanished.

So there I lay, in the dark, unable to move because any shift in my placement could've caused one of the hundreds of needles in my body to be driven in deeper and bring about more agonising pain. I was a hostage.

Wait! Bad choice of words — not a *hostage* ... As I said, Dr Nespith was an extremely charming and friendly man. I am not a racist. But I certainly felt like I was a hostage of some sort, someone who had been left in his cell to dwell on whether he should continue withholding important information from his captors. I would've felt this way if Dr Nespith had been Australian, Chinese, American or any race, creed or colour, let me say. It just so happened he was Iranian. Okay?

So anyway, there I lay in the dark, feeling like I was in an extremely non-racist hostage situation. It was very bizarre. What was I to do?

At this point let me add that if I ever were in a real hostage-torture situation, I'd give up every secret I had at the very first needle. It wouldn't take much. By needle four I'd be making up secrets. And as that final needle entered my scalp, I'd renounce my heritage and pledge allegiance to whatever group was holding me. These things *really* hurt.

Lying in the darkness I began to wonder if my liver and lungs had finally started to chat. Wasn't that the point of this whole exercise? I couldn't hear them talking, but I imagined how the conversation might've gone ...

'*So, it's been a while, eh Liver?*'

'*Sure has, Lungs. What've you been up to?*'

'*Oh, same ol' same ol'. Expanding, contracting — it's what I do.*'

'*Uh-huh.*'

'*And you?*'

'*Well, you know, my function is quite an important one ...*'

'*Are you saying mine isn't? Do you know how important* air *is, Liver?*'

'*Hey, I wasn't saying that. I was just saying that my job's pretty hard and —*'

'*Fuck, you always think you're so amazing! You think you're the most important part of the body and that everything revolves around you!*'

'*Oh, you think it revolves around* you, *do you?*'

'*I'm just saying that what I do is pretty damn important, pal!*'

'*Hey, hey, hey,*' interjects the heart. '*Can't we all just love one another?*'

'*Oh, fuck off, Heart!!*' they'd both yell in unison.

And within minutes they would all be back to where they'd started, with the heart in tears and the liver and lungs into their umpteenth year of non-communication.

Suddenly, the lights came on.

'Ow are you feeling, Misser Troy?' Dr Nespith asked with a newfound smile.

'Uh, weird,' I replied. 'How long have I been lying here?'

'Oh, about fizteen minutes. Not too long. It iz good, yez?'

'I guess,' I said, not really knowing how I should've been feeling. Had I fallen asleep at some stage? Was I healed, destined to never sweat profusely again? Would I bleed to death once all these needles were removed? I had so many questions.

'I vill take out ze needlez and we shall talk about ze next stepz,' Dr Nespith informed me, his accent seemingly more pronounced than ever before.

To be honest, the removal of the needles didn't hurt very much at all. The ones in my hands and on my head had been frighteningly painful during the previous fifteen minutes, and I was damn happy to be finally rid of them.

'You may take ze zeat again,' said the doctor once the removal process was complete.

I moved over to the chair as he revealed a plastic jar containing a concoction of herbs that he must've been blending for the duration of my period of light deprivation.

'What I ave made ere iz a mixture of herbs zat you must drink every day for ze next two weeks before you come back to zee me and we do zis again.'

Oh, I got it. This would be a 'process'. There was to be no instant cure, just an ongoing series of meetings until I'd paid this man enough money to buy himself a respectable living room. I knew how these things worked.

Dr Nespith continued. 'It vill taste yucky and your mouth vill not like it. But you must drink the mixture az it vill help you a lot, okay?' He was noticeably excited now. Perhaps he was curious to see if I'd actually drink his weird concoction of disgusting herbs.

'Sure,' I replied, clearly lying and desperate to get out of there. He must've sensed this.

'Zo, shall ve book you in for two veeks time now?' At this, he opened his diary to another empty Saturday.

'You know,' I began desperately, 'I'm not sure what I have on that Saturday, or over the next few weeks. Let me go home and check my diary and I'll call back when I know I'm free.'

He looked nervous. 'Vell, perhaps a tentative booking, zen? Shall ve say, Zaturday at ten?'

This was awkward.

'Yeah ... look, I'll call you, okay?' I repeated, sounding like a man who'd just had a bad first date.

'Oh. Okay.' He seemed almost heartbroken. 'Zen for now it iz yust zeventy dollarz. Do you ave cash?'

'Yes,' I said with a sigh and paid the man for the pain I'd endured. His heartbreak changed to joy very quickly.

As I was leaving I noticed another poor soul sitting nervously in the house's living/waiting room. I shook my head in her direction and motioned with my eyes for her to make a run for it, but I think I may've come across as a madman who'd come here for some sort of counselling. She would have to discover the truth for herself. You can't save them all.

Two days later I remembered to try the potion that Dr Nespith had given me and discovered it to be even yuckier than he'd promised. 'Fucking horrendous' would've described it better. It went straight in the bin.

Sadly, a week later I found myself drenched in sweat as the usual water torture took place throughout my body. But this time I simply transported my mind back to that even more unpleasant experience with the agonising needles and the horrific drink that followed, and realised that being frustrated and wet wasn't all that bad in comparison. Perhaps the work of Dr Nespith had been successful — as a deterrent of sorts. For although I still pour with sweat to this very day, I know that enduring a hostage situation round at my friendly neighbourhood acupuncturist's house sucks a whole lot more.

# 9
# TESTES, 100%

Sometimes life hands you an affirmation of your own personal perfection in the most unexpected way. One of my moments of greatness occurred on an extraordinary day when two men I had never previously met fondled my balls.

Please, allow me to explain.

For around a week I'd been experiencing an awkward sensation in the close vicinity of my right testicle. I say 'in the close vicinity' because, for the life of me, I was unable to establish the exact locale of this dull ache. It could've been in my upper thigh or groin, radiating to incorporate the right-hand nut, or it might've been the plum itself — I was unsure. The pain I felt is difficult to explain. It wasn't sharp and brutal; rather, it felt as if a tennis ball had whisked past my undercarriage and lightly clipped the right acorn on its way through.

Have you ever had a grazed bollock, gents? It's almost as painful as a swift kick to the entire set of goolies, but in a more mysterious way. The sickness that rises in your stomach after a gonad clash is exactly the same as that after a mere graze — it's just that the testicle itself isn't directly damaged.

No male likes the constant sensation that something isn't right with one of his man-eggs, so there was only one thing for it.

That being to sit quietly in my office chair all day, squirming and shifting uncomfortably until the pain subsided. Frustratingly, it didn't. In fact, it was getting worse.

To my mild embarrassment, a young female co-worker was the first to notice my discomfort and asked if I was okay.

'Uh, yeah,' I replied. 'Just a weird thing ... I think it's my groin.'

I am convinced that when I'm in a weakened physical condition I am also light of mind. Who, in their right mental state, tells an attractive female colleague that their groin is 'weird'? Not much of a pick-up line, let alone a topic of conversation that anyone would wish to join in on.

'Maybe you should go and see a doctor,' she suggested.

'Oh, it'll be fine. It's just a ... thing.' As I spoke, I mentally adjusted my underpants to loosen their elastic hold on my nuggets.

'Really? You wouldn't want it to drop off!' came her startling reply.

To all the women reading this, let me point out what an utterly brilliant line that was. If you ever want a man to go to a doctor regarding his man-parts but he won't go due to embarrassment, inform him of the potential for those parts to simply 'drop off'. While I've never heard of a man's meat and two veg simply falling off the plate, the mere notion is enough to make any male seek a medical appointment immediately and have someone inspect his bits for the slightest chance of droppage.

So there I was, an hour later, sitting in the waiting room of the local medical centre, about to expose my giggle-berries to an unsuspecting practitioner. Fantastic. Nothing awkward about that, is there?

The doctor welcomed me in and sat me down after a formal introduction. I promptly forgot his name, as I knew I'd never be seeing him again. It's just my nature.

I explained the reason for my visit in vague and mysterious terms and within seconds my trousers were around my knees and the man had his fingers on my pods. He seemed so keen to get his hands on them, I was almost suspicious. (Mind you, they are glorious.)

After a quick fondle and a peek, the doctor informed me that he had absolutely no idea what was wrong, and I would need to have an ultrasound before he could pass any further judgment on my pebbles.

'An ultrasound?' I asked, already knowing what an ultrasound was but keen to keep him engaged in conversation, lest he go back to rummaging around my parts.

'Yes, to see that everything is okay down there. I mean, there's a chance that it's simply a pulled ligament in your thigh and the pain is displaced, but it's best to be sure.'

Best to be sure so that things don't fall off, I recalled.

The doctor wrote me out a referral and sent me on my nervous way to another medical centre, which was in no way nearby, to display my marbles to a second unsuspecting quack. Perhaps they were so wonderful he wanted to share the joy around. I assumed so.

After an expensive and nasally overwhelming cab ride to the next venue, I shuffled to the counter and was greeted by a guy called Tim, who politely advised me that he'd be the one handling my guy-pouch this afternoon. He guided me into a dimly lit room and, quite unromantically, explained the procedure that was about to take place.

'Now Troy, what I'll get you to do is drop your pants to your knees and hop up on the bed here, and then I'll place this electronic device on your scrotum. Don't worry, it won't hurt, but it will feel a little cold as I have to apply a gel to it.'

'Gel?' I enquired. 'Hey, when you're done, maybe we can style the hair down there too?'

Tim didn't find me amusing at all. In the silence that followed, I slowly dropped my strides and climbed onto the bed. Tim handed me some lengths of paper towel, which he had twisted and contorted into an origami hammock. He then, ever so casually, picked up my wang and placed it in the paper pouch, briefly showing me how to hold it back using the contorted towel. It was like restraining a wild bull behind the gates at a rodeo.

'Whoa! Down, big fella!' I joked.

I wish I hadn't, though, because Tim was looking even less amused than before. I guess he wasn't too happy in his job, poor guy.

So now, with my member in its paper restraints, Tim had a bird's-eye view of my testicles in all their rotund, hirsute glory. He rubbed some lube on an electrified metal *deely* (that's medical terminology, so you might not understand it) and placed said *deely* directly onto my nuts. Yowser!

Using the array of high-tech gadgets connected to the *deely*, Tim proceeded to take some glorious pictures of my fruit bowl from the inside. He did a few lazy circles of the area, like a hoon in a Valiant out the back of a suburban milk bar, before handing me some more towelling to wipe the slippery gel off myself. (I'm sorry, but it had to be said.)

Next, I played the waiting game. Thirty full minutes would pass before I could know the fate of my loins and, to be honest, this was when the reality of the situation set in. For approximately twenty-five of those thirty minutes, I sat there in silence, growing more and more concerned at the possible outcome of the tests on my testes. There was every chance that Tim would discover some sort of testicular cancer, infertility or general abnormality of some description. To be honest, the thought of this had me extremely distressed.

So when he finally reappeared from the developing room, I frantically searched his face for any signs of despair on behalf of my lower ornaments. He approached me with an air of nonchalance, handed me some x-rays and his written appraisal, before promptly disappearing without comment back into his dimly lit room. Not a word.

Without hesitation, I ripped open the envelope and scanned the results. They read as follows: BOTH TESTES ARE OF NORMAL SIZE AND ECHO PATTERN. TESTES, 100 PER CENT.

*Excellent!* My sigh of relief could be heard several streets over.

But let me dwell on a couple of things here for a moment. Firstly, 'normal size'? They are much bigger than normal size, thank you very much. Clearly Tim had become jaded in his profession and decided to take it out on me. Perhaps he was just jealous of my manhood.

Secondly, what did he mean by 'echo pattern'? At no point did Dr Tim hold up my penis like a microphone and yell into it to achieve a result. Had he done so, he might very well have encountered the gloriously resounding echo of my plum chambers; but since he hadn't, I was left to assume that he wasn't really doing his job properly.

Tim, I hope you've started taking a little more pride in your work, my friend.

THIS IS AN ESSENTIALLY NORMAL SCROTAL ULTRASOUND, the report went on, OTHER THAN THE PATIENT POSSESSING A TRULY IMPRESSIVE-SIZED PENIS. (I may've embellished that second part.)

The point here was that my tea-bags were fine. No, they were more than fine, they were 100 per cent — I had it in writing. A shining example of scrotal perfection housed right here in my pants. I felt like showing everyone.

And with the knowledge that my knapsack was without flaw, I was later informed that the dull ache *was* merely the displaced pain of a ligament injury, as the previous doctor had assumed. An ache, I might add, that soon went away ... on its own. Quite naturally.

As I wrote at the start of this chapter, there is nothing like life's foibles to hand you an affirmation of your own personal perfection — and when it does, you should shout it from the rooftops. So, as you drive home today, or while you're lying in your bed at night, keep an ear out for my voice being carried on the wind. You'll know it's me, for I'll be the one on the roof of my apartment block, proudly yelling at the top of my lungs:

*'Testes — 100 per cent!'*

# 10
# THE BURNING
## (OR: SO THIS IS WHAT HELL FEELS LIKE)

On Christmas Eve one year, filled with the joy and free-flowing liquids of the festive season, while also celebrating my birthday, I somehow managed to convince a female acquaintance that kissing me would be one of the most cherished gifts she could offer to express her friendship. Either that or an iPod. With the price of iPods still similar to that of a small car back then — yet capable of so very much more, I might add — she took the kissing option.

But here's the thing … At some stage during the drunken exchange of spit that evening, she casually referred to an annoying bump above her lip. 'I think I'm getting a pimple,' she commented in a boozy slur.

*Whatever*, I thought.

As nonchalant as I was at the time, so began a week of my life that would go on to become a saga of epic proportions.

## 25 December — Merry bloody Christmas to you too

What is normally a day for celebration and unbridled happiness for many religious families and communities throughout the world began with fear and horror for me that year. I awoke with a mild hangover and what could only be described as freakishly giant, cartoon lips. Overnight, somewhere between the time my drunken mouth left hers and the light of morning, my lips became inflated like rubber life-rafts and now had a mild burning sensation similar to when you kiss a hot barbecue in summer. (Don't try it, just understand it.)

Due at my parents' place for the traditional festivities in less than an hour, I immediately panicked and phoned my mother. 'Mum!' I mumbled through my gargantuan mouth-futons. 'My lips are swollen and they're burning. I'm freaking out and I don't know what to do!'

'Calm down,' she replied. 'Now, what happened? Did you kiss someone you shouldn't have?'

'Um ...' My pause gave me away, but I continued to play dumb. 'No! I just — I woke up like this.' Jeez, even I wasn't buying it. Uwe Boll films had more convincing dialogue than this.

'Well, don't worry about it. It's probably only an allergic reaction to something you ate yesterday,' she said. 'Come over and I'll take a look. You'll be fine. It's Christmas!'

And with that gesture of seasonal good cheer, she hung up and went about her usual preparations of chilling wine and uncorking champagne. What can I say? — my family loves Christmas.

I sat down on my bed and stared into the mirrored wardrobe, prodding and poking at my lips like they were a strange new alien life form that had attached itself to my face in order to feed and, eventually, take over the world. I'd seen this happen in movies a million times.

What occurred next I simply cannot explain. I mean, I will for the purposes of you, the reader — but it defies any logic or medical science that I'm aware of. Quite simply, over the next half-hour or so, everything healed. By the time I arrived at my parents' house, my lips had returned to their normal size and the burning had subsided. Nothing on this planet could've conspired to make me look more neurotic in front of my mum than this. This ... *nothingness*.

On hearing my car door close out in the street with her finely tuned ears, Mum raced out to the kerb to greet me and study the medical condition I'd described so frantically down the phone. 'Oh Troy, you had me so worried — and there's nothing there!' she exclaimed. 'What are you so worried about? You look perfectly normal.'

'Well, it's gone now. But it *was* there. And it was really bad. And—'

'It's all in your head, darling! You've always had a thing about the way you look.'

Had I? Well, if I hadn't before I certainly did now.

'Come inside and have a glass of champagne. It's Christmas!' Mum announced again as though I had already forgotten.

Merrily, the day rolled on. Celebrations were had, gifts were exchanged and alcohol was consumed, albeit cautiously by me, until everyone was too exhausted to continue.

Tired and relieved, I departed my parents' abode and headed for the airport. It had become a tradition of mine each year to catch a flight up to Queensland's Sunshine Coast and unwind for two weeks while the company I worked for closed down over the Christmas break. This would be the fourth year in a row I'd spend at this location, but the first time in my life I would visit a doctor interstate.

Actually, not just one doctor, but three. Two of whom were total idiots.

## 26 December — Boxing Day in my boxer shorts

When I went to bed that night of the 25th, I was in a different state. Not just mentally relaxed and mildly intoxicated, but also in a completely different part of Australia. Waking up in the same place you crashed out in would normally be a good thing; however, on drifting out of sleep that Boxing Day morning, I immediately wanted to be back at home.

Why?

The *burning*.

The burning in my lips had mysteriously returned, the swelling mildly present as well. But now, in a wonderful turn of events, there seemed to be a touch of burning around the groin area. That's right — burning around my groin.

As any other rational adult would, I completely freaked out and began running around the room like a psychopathic escapee. *How could this have happened to me?* I thought. *I'm a good person — I only kissed the girl! What has she given me?* My reaction made perfect sense: scream at the walls, run around in a panic, look at every body part in the mirror, and become increasingly alarmed at every imperfection I could find. The problem was, I couldn't find any. (Well, not in the region I was most concerned about, anyway.)

My groin was only a little warm, like a mild case of sunburn, but, having not exposed it to sun for many, many years, I knew that something wasn't right. And I'd expected to find some sort of rash or at least a bump of some nature, but there was absolutely nothing. No signs of devastation whatsoever. What to do, what to do?

*Think logically*, I thought illogically. *Find an internet café and work out what this is!* Genius.

I threw on some shorts and a pair of thongs and raced to the nearest venue that had an 'e' logo on the door. For $3 I could have forty minutes' worth of research time. Surely that would be more than enough to diagnose my new, clearly fatal, disease.

Search: 'burning sensation on lips, groin and thighs'. Result: 157,000,000 entries. Yikes. Maybe forty minutes wouldn't be quite enough.

I clicked on the first entry, which immediately concluded that I had some form of vaginal itching. Oh, perhaps not ... Try again. The next site appeared to confirm that I had one of several sexually transmitted diseases currently travelling around the planet on the wild merry-go-round of lust. But there was no way to verify exactly what I was suffering from, as so many of these diseases had similar symptoms, yet none of them completely matched mine in all its forms. Only one mentioned swollen, burning lips, for instance.

This website — which, it must be said, looked like nothing more than a teenagers' blog page — explained something I hadn't even considered. It stated that a weird sensation in the lips could be the first sign of a cold sore, and that a cold sore is a variation of the herpes virus; in addition, if touched, a cold sore can be transferred to the groin area and change into the other type of herpes ... You know, the type no one wants. Ever.

So, could that pimple on the face of the girl I'd kissed have actually been a cold sore? Could I have caught it and somehow transferred it downstairs into my trousers? Surely not.

One thing was clear: if I wanted to know the truth, I was going to have to see a real doctor. There was no woman around to send me on my way, but the eternal maternal voice of my mother was rattling around inside my head, and that was enough for me. Besides, these symptoms had all been caused by a woman, I assumed, so that was the same as being sent to a doctor by one, in a round-about kind of way.

With twenty-three minutes left of internet time and no way of simply logging off until it had counted down, I surfed across sites I had very little or no interest in until the final seconds lapsed and the computer's search history was immediately erased. If only the burning could've been erased that easily.

Outside the café I found a tourist information kiosk and enquired as to the whereabouts of the nearest medical centre.

The well-tanned woman running the kiosk produced a local phone directory and began flipping through the pages frantically. After a long and exhaustive search, she pointed down the street to a glass building approximately 50 metres away. You had to wonder how she'd never noticed it before.

I made my way in there and was instantly greeted with fevered excitement by the elderly receptionist, who seemed thrilled to have a new customer to add to the four already scattered around the waiting room. She took down my details and asked me to have a seat, speaking loudly and briskly like a school mistress on speed. It was friendly and frightening all at once.

After the shuffling of several folders and plenty of loud, brisk telephone conversations with what seemed to be family and friends, the aged receptionist informed me I could walk down the short hallway to Dr Reed's office, as he was ready to see me now. I wondered how ready for this he was.

Dr Reed was old too. Not simply elderly, but ridiculously, almost hilariously, old. There was a good chance he had once been Moses' personal physician or even a vet during the Jurassic Period. Straight away I felt a sense of unease.

'Hello there, I'm Dr Reed. How are you today?' he began.

'I'm fine, thanks,' I replied automatically, before realising the inaccuracy of my response.

'What seems to be the problem?'

'Well … I was with this girl,' I started, nervously. The nervousness wasn't due to the nature of the conversation, but mostly because Dr Reed hadn't bothered to close his door after welcoming me in. The hallway was short and I had already overheard other patients discussing their ailments while I'd been waiting.

'Go on,' he said sternly.

'Well, it was my birthday and, um, I met a girl …' I was

whispering at this point. 'And there was some ... er, well, *oral behaviours ...*'

I had never, and have never since, referred to kissing as 'oral behaviours', but they were the words that came out of my tingling, overwrought mouth. I think I was trying to sound medical within those medical surrounds. I continued.

'And, well, now my lips are burning really, really badly and I think I might've caught something from, er ... her.' Christ, that was awkward. Surely, 'I kissed a girl' would've done the job much more succinctly.

'Your lips burn, you say?'

'Yes. Hotly,' came my ludicrous reply.

'Well, that doesn't sound like an STD. Are there any other symptoms?'

I was shocked. How could it not have been an STD? I kissed a girl and now my lips were on fire. It was *definitely* an STD. This man didn't know anything.

'Um, there's also a slight burning around my groin and thighs,' I added, to emphasise the fact that I knew more about this problem than he did.

'No, that's probably not there. I'm sure it's mostly in your mind,' he announced without a shred of evidence.

*In my mind? No sir, it's mostly in my pants!* That's what I wanted to respond with. Sadly, I didn't. 'In my mind? What do you mean?' was my honest response.

'Well, you have burning on your lips and you've decided it's an STD, so you're simply transferring the pain mentally because you feel that this is where it should be. Don't worry about that, let's worry about your lips. Because it's not an STD.'

'It's not?'

'No, it's not. Well, none that I know of, anyway,' he said, quite matter-of-factly.

This man had been around since the dawn of time. I assumed he would've known them all.

'Have you eaten any fish or berries lately that you may have had a reaction to?' the good doctor enquired.

'No. None.'

'What about lip balms — ChapStick, that sort of thing — do you use anything like that?'

'No. Nothing at all,' I replied, building the case in my mind that it was still definitely an STD.

'Hmm,' he hummed thoughtfully. 'It seems we have a mystery on our hands.'

On our lips, more like it. Everything he did made me want to cry out: *I have a fucking STD! Just tell me what it is and I can begin the healing process or learn how to deal with it for the rest of my life. Work it out, doc!* But instead I sat there looking quizzical and mystified as Dr Reed stared off into space, racking his brains for the blatantly obvious answer.

'Wait a minute!' He'd broken the silence at last. 'Have you used any sort of mouthwash recently?'

He'd hit on something there. 'Uh, yes. Yes, I did. On Christmas Eve.' I recalled the lazy use of mouthwash to 'clean my teeth' after stumbling home from the pub that same night. I hadn't used a mouthwash for months before then, nor afterwards. Just that one moment.

'Well, that's it! I see it all the time.'

If he saw it all the time, then how come it took him so long to figure it out, eh? Surely that would've been the first conclusion he'd reach every time. This was becoming farcical!

'I don't understand,' I said.

'Well, those mouthwashes are the worst things around for your mouth. They clean out all the bacteria — but not only the bad bacteria, the good bacteria as well.'

'There's *good* bacteria?'

'Of course! And it fights off infections and the like. But the mouthwash you've used has killed off all the good bacteria and now you have an infection. It's so simple. Here, I'll give you some tablets to take and it will clear everything up by tomorrow. You go and pour that mouthwash down the drain — it's the worst thing on the market!'

The offending mouthwash was all the way back in another state, but I didn't have the heart to tell him. 'But what about my ... *thing*?' I asked quietly, noting again that the door was wide open.

'Oh, I told you — it's all in your head. You'll be fine. Relax!' With that, Dr Reed threw some nondescript tablets into an envelope and handed it to me while ushering me out through the ever-open door.

I fixed up my bill with the loud receptionist and hastily made my retreat, still unsure whether I'd been handed the cure or merely a distraction. Perhaps the doctor was phoning around his medical colleagues to see if they had any idea what could've been causing this burning mystery.

Whatever had just happened, my only option right now was to go with it. A block from the medical centre, I ripped open the envelope and threw two tablets down my throat so that the healing could begin. Something inside me knew, however, that all was still not right with the world.

## 27 December — This isn't good

At around 3am I awoke in what can only be described as agony. Pure, burning agony. My groin and thighs had been consumed by such fire and heat that I was ripped from my sleep to begin cursing the wretched doctor who, a mere seventeen hours before, had advised me that it was all in my head.

I leapt from the bed and ran into the bathroom to get a close look at the region and self-diagnose once more. Throwing on the light switch, I thrust my underwear to my ankles and waited with frustration for my eyes to adjust to the sudden visual intrusion of brightness in my retinas.

Waiting.

Waiting.

Freaking out.

Waiting.

When my eyes had finally found their focus, I hunched over as far as I could and peered more closely at my manhood than I ever had in my life. Christ, it's not an attractive part of the body, is it? No wonder we keep it covered up until the last minute with women.

But there it was, unchanged from the days, weeks or months before, resting in my hand like it was still sound asleep, just as the rest of me should've been. I turned it like a sausage on a grill and contorted it every which way I could to see the underside and its surrounds — all to no avail. I couldn't find anything wrong with it at all.

But the burning was now so strong that there was no way this could simply have been in my head. The heat radiating from my lap could've warmed a small hut in winter. It was almost unbearable. And it was sore too. It actually felt as though I'd wounded my groin, yet there was no wound to be found. The situation defied all logic, so there was nothing left to do but pray and remain confused.

All this and it was only 3 o'clock in the morning. I'd have to wait another six hours before I could show my lack of symptoms to the doctor again and beg him to rethink his diagnosis.

Waiting.

Waiting.

Freaking out.

Checking the appendage and general region again for change.

No change.

Freaking out.

Waiting.

Waiting.

This was how the hours unfolded. I must've checked myself for any sort of change at least thirty times during those terrifying six hours, so that by the time I was seated in the medical centre's waiting room, my manhood was probably red raw from simple over-handling.

'What are you doing back here?' yelled the receptionist, unnecessarily loudly.

'I need to see the doctor again, please.'

'But you were in here yesterday!' she screeched with delight.

'Er ... yes. Yes, I was. I need to see him again. *Please.*' I don't know why I was now pleading with her. She could hardly deny my request. I mean, there's no law against seeing a doctor two days in a row, is there?

'Well, Dr Reed isn't here today. You'll have to see Dr Hart,' she told me sternly.

Anyone would be fine, and I thanked her humbly. Then I made my way over to one of the empty chairs and sat there, uncomfortably, to await my fate.

Somehow, three patients had managed to make it into the waiting room before me, so naturally they were the first to be served by Dr Hart. Since I had arrived here bang on opening time, according to the sign on the door, I could only imagine there'd been an early-morning queue of three people truly desperate to gain entry to this medical centre. I understood their urgency. Perhaps they'd kissed the same girl that I had.

I sat there and waited while listening to each of their diagnoses from Dr Hart, who seemed to have the same habit of not closing his office door as Dr Reed. Surely this open-door policy jeopardised the doctor–patient confidentiality arrangement, no? All I cared about right now, though, was stopping the burning. I had a bushfire in my pants, and I was none too happy about what could've been causing it.

After what seemed like an eternity, Dr Hart appeared and led me into his office. I turned and reached for the door, to shut it behind me, but he beat me to it.

'Don't worry about that, mate,' he said, swinging his hand limply off the door and closing it by a mere 5 centimetres. Alas, this meant it was still wide open and any movement from me now to shut it properly would've appeared alarmingly neurotic.

Dr Hart was a fat man. Not obese, but clearly not someone with a penchant for exercise or a healthy diet. How could this bloke, knowing everything I assumed he did about the human body, allow his own to become such a mess? From my point of view, this did not instil great confidence in his abilities. The best description I can give of Dr Hart is to say that he strongly resembled Les Patterson, without the charm.

'So, tell me what's wrong, mate.'

I took a deep breath. 'Well, on Christmas Eve I kissed this girl and then my lips started burning, so I came in here yesterday and the doctor told me it was from mouthwash and he gave me some tablets. But then last night my groin and thighs started burning and now it's really burning a lot, and I think I may have contracted an STD of some sort — but I really don't know how. So I was hoping you could tell me.'

'Oral sex?' He sounded almost disgusted.

I tilted my head, a little stunned by what he'd said. 'No ... not oral sex. There was only kissing. Unless you *mean* kissing, do you? Is kissing a type of oral sex?' I was nervous now. I hadn't mentioned oral sex, so why was he jumping to that conclusion?

'Mate, it's fine. How are your lips? Are they still burning?'

'Not so much,' I replied. 'But I can't really tell because all I can focus on is this heat coming off my groin. It's like a really bad case of sunburn, but I've never had it out in the sun.'

'All right then, mate. Why don't you take your pants down and show me your bits?' he said loudly and bluntly.

Charming. Part of this put me a little more at ease, however — I liked his directness. Dr Hart was cutting through the bullshit and getting on with the job at hand. I respected that. Now, if he could just have done it a little more quietly and with the door closed, I'd have been a whole lot happier.

With some trepidation, I dropped my trousers. I expected him to look at my parts, declare that I had an incurable STD and send me on my way, still burning. But, much to my surprise, he fumbled with my nether-region for a few seconds before telling me to pull up my pants and take a seat again. Surely this could only have meant something serious — you never hear anyone say 'Take a seat' if the news is good ...

'Well, there's nothing wrong with your dick, mate,' Dr Hart told me and whoever was listening in a few metres down the hall.

'But the whole area is on *fire*!' I cried.

'Yeah, I can't really explain that. Basically, if you had an STD of some kind, then I should be able to see some spots or something similar. But I can't. And besides, if you only kissed the girl, it wouldn't affect your dick. There's nothing there.'

'Well, there's *something* there. I can feel it burning. Is there any sort of explanation you can give me?'

'Look, if you want to do a blood and urine test then I can arrange for that, and that should make it perfectly clear if there's anything sexually transmitted in your system. Do you want to do that?'

*Hell, yeah!* I almost cheered. I'd done enough research the day before to know that once I had the official diagnosis, many STDs could be cured by antibiotics. Sure, many couldn't, but they could at least be managed. Whatever — as long as it put an end to the burning.

'How long will it take to get the results?' I asked desperately.

'Oh, about three days.'

'*Three days*? What am I meant to do in the meantime?' I gasped.

'Well, I can prescribe you an antibiotic that will cure things like chlamydia and gonorrhoea, in case you've picked those up from somewhere else. Other than that — wait.'

I accepted his offer of an antibiotic prescription, just in case, and promptly made another booking for three days' time to pick up the results once I'd done the tests. The others in the waiting room shuffled nervously in their chairs as I wandered past them towards the door. No doubt they'd heard about the burning.

Across the road from the medical centre in a public toilet cubicle, while urinating in a plastic cup, I was once again with my trousers around my ankles inspecting my groin for spots or bumps, as though they had merely decided to wait to appear until I was out of view of my doctor. You know, like an infected version of Harvey the Rabbit. There was still nothing there other than the regular male appendage, and it made me angry. It wasn't that I actually wanted to have an STD, of course; I simply needed a reason for the pain I was in.

A cup of urine later and I was in a new part of the medical centre, giving blood to an expressionless nurse who obviously wasn't too keen on any sort of general conversation.

'So, how much blood do I have to give?' I tried.

'Just be still. It'll be over in a minute.'

I took it that it was my tongue she wanted to be 'still', but I was having none of it. If she was going to drain my very life source from me, the least I expected was a little bit of a chat to go with it. 'Uh … how long does it take for the results to come back, nurse?'

I already knew the answer to this question and had even booked the appointment accordingly, but I really wanted this woman to open up a little.

'Your doctor would've told you that,' she responded tersely.

'Oh, yeah. Thanks.'

And that was that. She was done with her bloody task and I was out of there like a shot. The less time I spent with these people, the better.

Now, I ask you, what would you do with three days to spare, a strong heat sensation in your groin and thighs, and a half-depleted bank account thanks to a wide array of useless but expensive consultations, tablets and tests? Me, I went to the beach.

Over the many years of injuries and illnesses I'd endured thus far, there was a saying I routinely heard fall from my mother's lips: 'Salt water cures everything.' I didn't think this could be entirely true, as I'd never heard of anyone with cancer, a heart condition or even hiccups being cured after a quick dip at the nearest beach, but right now I was willing to try pretty much anything. Plus, I'd just flown up to one of the most beautiful beaches on the planet for two weeks of relaxation and tanning. I was determined to soak in a little bit of this goodness while I was here.

I raced back to the apartment and threw off all my infected clothes, replacing them with a pair of boardshorts and a resolve to cure whatever was going on with my bollocks. I made sure not to wear any underwear at this point, as I wanted to be positive that the salt water was getting right onto the area in all its miraculous, healing glory.

Moments later I was waist-deep in the great blue ocean and absolutely loving the feeling of cool water on my hot nether-region. I sighed with relief and genuinely expected to hear the hissing sound of steam as the sea caressed my plums. It was a pure delight ... for a few measly moments.

Gradually the joy and relief gave way to anger and disappointment as my body adjusted to the cool water temperature and began to inform me that the sunburn sensation was still very much present, even underwater. *Fuck*.

Looking around at the other swimmers frolicking in the ocean and laughing with one another, I immediately began to hate them. Then, in a split second, I was overcome with the fear that maybe these people knew what I was experiencing here in the smooth blue depths ... Had they been in the waiting room of the medical centre while my diagnosis was loudly announced by the doctor? Could it be that word had been spread across the entire beach by concerned citizens who didn't want the neighbouring state's mysterious burning disease cultivating on any of the local residents? If not, then why was everyone staring at me?

*Blurghghbggharh uhblububublphh blaarghupupa.*

Let me tell you two things I learned in that very brief moment:

1. Nobody knows about the burning sensation in your pants and, even if they did, most of them don't give a flying fuck. Everyone has their own problems to deal with, and if you think they care about yours, you're paranoid and delusional. Snap out of it.

2. Nothing helps you snap out of it faster than a large, unexpected wave hitting you on the head and washing you 50 metres underwater back to shore. Never turn your back on the ocean.

The reason everyone had been looking at me was because I was standing there staring at them as one of the day's biggest waves crept up behind me to slap me in the head. No doubt many people had foreseen the hilarity that was about to ensue and had stopped to take a look. Funny for them, I guess, but not for me.

I picked myself up out of the ankle-deep water to the sound of children sniggering in the shallows, pulled a large piece of seaweed out of my tangled hair and lumbered back to my towel, with the heat of my groin still reminding me that this day wasn't about to get better any time soon. Salt water doesn't cure everything. Sometimes it simply creates more problems.

## 28 December — Feeling hot, hot, hot (another reason to hate that song)

The day before had not gone well. After the wipeout episode, I spent the majority of it indoors watching television, waiting for my groin and thighs to change appearance. Every thirty minutes I checked thoroughly and found no trace of damage. It was driving me insane. And the night-time was even worse.

Come morning, having hardly slept a wink in the past forty-eight hours, my ability to accept that this was merely a 'mystery' was fading fast. So, throwing on some loose-fitting clothes under the misconception that perhaps the closeness of the fabric might be partly to blame, I left my abode at 8:30am, determined to find a doctor who knew what he was doing.

I recalled hearing Dr Hart's loud-voiced receptionist informing someone that there was another medical centre down the road, at the end of the block. So that was where I was headed now. I walked awkwardly to this new destination and came across a large sign reading: SKIN CANCER CLINIC AND FITNESS CENTRE.

It sounded medical-ish, though hardly wang-related. Nor would it have been embarrassing had I not been so stupid as to ask the lycra-clad girl at the front desk if the area behind her with treadmills and weight-lifting equipment in was a medical centre.

'Uh, no. This is a gym,' she replied. 'The medical centre is across the road.' I could've sworn she followed these directions with the word 'moron' muttered under her breath, but I'll give her the benefit of the doubt.

Across the road was the largest, clearest, brightest sign for a medical centre I had ever seen. Surely they hadn't just installed it while I was making an arse of myself over at the gym, had they? How I missed that sign before, I'll never know.

This medical centre 'down the road, at the end of the block' was in stark contrast to the one I had become familiar with over the past few days. It was as quiet as a library. The receptionist spoke in a barely audible whisper and there were no other patients in the waiting room. I liked this place. As edgy as I was about the burning mystery in my pants, I felt a mild calm sweep over me as I sat there waiting for a doctor to appear. The general aura of this venue was clearly designed with a sick patient in mind and I wished I'd come here from the start.

After a few moments of anxious waiting, the doctor appeared. He was charming, calm and, although he struggled a little with the English language, I knew from the moment he turned to shut the door behind us that he would hold the answer to all my troubles. This guy really knew his business.

I told the doctor, in my usual, irrational blurb, about the fire down below and let him have a quick fondle of my junk while I waited for the death sentence to be read.

He smiled. 'You calm down and be fine,' he said peacefully.

'What? How will it be fine?'

'You have the prostatitis. I give you antibiotics and it will all clear up. It's all fine.'

'I have the prostatitis?' I blurted, not even knowing what that was. 'I'm pretty sure I have AIDS or something. How can you be so sure? How do you know it's this other thing?'

'I've seen this before. Not STD — no spots, no nothing. Not

AIDS. Not dying, only infection. Everything is being fine,' he told me calmly and confidently.

'Are you *sure?*'

'I'm sure. Relax.' He was almost laughing now.

I think I laughed a little as well, for the first time in what seemed like forever. The weight had been lifted off my shoulders and the pain even seemed to subside a touch. In one, calm, brief encounter, this man had allayed all my fears and torments and handed me a prescription for the cure. I think I was in love.

'Oh, and drink some cranberry juice to keep everything good,' he added as I walked out.

'Cranberry juice? You got it!' I yelled, proudly.

And with that, I was sorted. I bolted to the chemist like a man possessed and picked up my prescribed cure, before darting over to the supermarket and buying out their supply of cranberry juice. If cranberries made things 'good', then I was going to be fucking fantastic.

## 29 December — The wait continues

You'd think that by now everything would've been absolutely fine, wouldn't you? I mean, I'd had a confident diagnosis, I had the tablets to cure my condition and I was practically bathing in cranberry juice to ensure prolonged goodness — what could I possibly have had to worry about? The tests, that's what. Still looming in the back of my mind was the very real possibility that the good, calm doctor was actually wrong. I didn't want to think this, because I liked him the best, but only with time and my test results could I ever be sure.

Time. Fucking time.

So I ask you again, what do you do with days to wait and a still-burning crotch, even if you have the all-clear? Nothing but continue to freak out — and that's exactly what I did.

Waiting.
Waiting.
Freaking out.
Checking the appendage again for change.
No change.
Freaking out.
Waiting.
Waiting.

## 30 December — The wait continues to continue

Waiting.
Waiting.
Freaking out.
Checking the region again for change.
No change.
Freaking out.
Waiting.
Waiting.

## 31 December — Result!

Today, the final day of the year, was going to determine if my New Year would begin with celebration or not. I won't lie — I was fucking nervous. Dr Reed was the one who delivered the news.

'Well, how can I help you today?' the old man asked, not recognising me even remotely.

'Um ... I was in here a few days ago with some burning on my lips and —'

'Oh, yes. Has that gone away?' he interrupted.

'Yeah. But then things got a lot worse and my groin and thighs started burning furiously and it hasn't stopped at all.'

'Well, that's unrelated.'

'Er, sure — yet still very important to me. So forget the lip thing for now,' I pleaded.

'So now you think your groin and thighs are burning?'

'Hey, I *know* they're burning, but I don't know what's causing it. So I came in the day after I saw you and Dr Hart arranged for some blood tests, and he said they'd be back today,' I coaxed.

'Why don't you drop your pants and we'll have a look, shall we? Burning, you say?'

I honestly don't know if he heard anything I'd said about the blood tests. The expression on his face hinted at the possibility that his hearing aid might've been on the blink.

'Yeah, burning. But I'd also like to check the tests to see if they showed anything,' I said as I lowered my trousers.

'Well, we can do some tests, but it doesn't look like there's anything to be concerned about.'

'Listen,' I said in a raised voice while I did up my button fly, 'I have *had* tests. I am here for the results. I saw another doctor a couple of days ago who told me that I have prostatitis, and he's given me antibiotics for it. So now I want to be sure.' I was desperate by this stage.

'Prostatitis? No, it's definitely not that,' he said, breaking my spirit completely.

'Well, what is it then?'

'Let's take a look at the test results and find out, shall we?' he suggested, in a rare moment of clarity, and began scanning the paperwork in front of him. 'Hmm ... everything here is normal. No STDs, no infections ... Perhaps it's all in your head.'

'You've got to be kidding me! My groin and thighs feel like they've been dipped in acid, and you're telling me it's all in my head? That can't be right!'

'Well, it's not an STD and there's nothing in your tests to indicate any sort of infection, so I would just try to ride it out until it goes away. Perhaps if you work it out you can tell me what it was!' he finished, laughing.

And that was that. Dr Reed sent me from his office more confused than when I'd walked in. My tests revealed nothing — for which I am sure I should've been grateful — but without any anomaly in the results, I was unable to work out what was causing my condition. Worse still, I was unable to cure it. Isn't that what doctors are meant to do?

I had no other choice than to continue with the belief that I had prostatitis and that the tablets I'd been given would cure it.

And honestly, after a few days it seemed like they had. There was no pain, no burning and no more stress. I still had a week left of my holiday in which to relax and unwind, so I took full advantage of my fresh-feeling groin and took in as many of the wonderful sights and sounds of the Sunshine Coast as my wallet could muster.

It was fantastic and my wang felt glorious again ... for now.

# 11
# THE BURNING RETURNING
## (OR: THIS HEAT IS DRIVING ME NUTS!)

About a month passed after those last pangs of flame had subsided from my groin, during which I almost completely forgot about the horrendous debacle that my Christmas holiday had become. It's amazing how quickly you can forget the agony and panic that had once wracked your brain when, at the time, they seemed like the only thing in the world that mattered. Sadly, ignorance can only remain bliss for so long.

## 3 February — Here we go again
I was lying on the couch watching TV, as is my wont, when I felt a very light, yet strangely familiar, burning sensation on the inside of my upper thigh. Right where the testicle meets the thigh. (Yeah, right in there. Can you feel it?)

Immediately I freaked out and began dreading the return of that raging beast that had plagued me not long before. Most of this freak-out involved little more than running a sort of internal dialogue of anger and fear. To be honest, I didn't even get up off the couch. As usual, I just hoped it would go away.

## 4 February — The power of hope and TV

My crotch and thighs were consumed. Not by the joyful caresses of a loving partner, but by the heat. What had started on the couch yesterday as a small, localised area of burn had now spread to cover the entire region again.

Manhood — check. Inner thighs — check. Outer thighs — check. Testicles — double check ... They were all there, covered in pain.

However, this particular 4th of February was a Sunday. Everyone knows Sundays are the laziest days in town. Most people would never name their child Sunday, because it would grow up to be obese and achieve absolutely nothing (unless it was a celebrity child). It's a given.

So, being a lazy Sunday, I parked my burning body down on the couch and watched an excessive amount of television to while away the hours. There was no point seeking out medical assistance. I had only one option: hope.

## 5 February — All hope is gone

Something in life that's never fun is having to call your mother to discuss your burning crotch. It's not a phone call I can recommend to any male. Apart from the awkwardness and the anxiety it causes your mum, such conversations leave you feeling like an evil child who's admitted to his mother that she raised him to be promiscuous. Don't ask me why, it just does. But I had to do something about the constant heat and pain. And calling my mum was certainly easier than, say, walking the three blocks from my office to the doctor's surgery.

'Mum, I have a terrible burning sensation in my groin and across my thighs,' I began, horrified as the words spilled forth from my mouth. 'I don't know what it is, but it's quite painful and I'm a little freaked out here. There's no rash, no marks, nothing — just the burning. Any ideas?'

'Sorry, I think you might have the wrong number,' came the voice in reply.

Okay, it didn't really, but I almost wished it had. I was not comfortable telling my mother about this situation at all.

'Well, darling,' she said, 'you should probably go and see a doctor about it. I have no idea what could cause that. Have you been with any strange women lately?'

How do you answer a question like that from your mother?! Any response is going to be a letdown. If I had been sleeping with 'strange women', then she'd have been bitterly disappointed by my behaviour. On the other hand, my not having engaged in sexual relations of any nature lately might leave her feeling as though she'd raised a less-than-sexually-successful son. I worry about things like this, hence my general lack of sleep.

'No, Mum,' I told her honestly. 'No strange women.'

'Then go and see a doctor and get it sorted out,' she replied, putting faith in modern medicine and its stated ability to diagnose any ailment correctly. History and experience, however, had taught me otherwise.

## 6 February — F***ing doctors

After enduring another night of flaming pain and hourly checks of my fiery bits, I woke up with a determination to get everything sorted out as soon as possible.

When my lunchbreak finally arrived at work, I headed straight to the local medical centre and begged feverishly to see the first available shaman. With an efficiency I hadn't experienced during my previous burning situation, the receptionist silently typed some details into her computer and asked me to take a seat in the waiting room. 'It won't be long,' she assured me.

Now, I'm not sure how this woman defined 'long' exactly, but I was certain that no man would ever measure up to her ideal. When it came to time, her 'It won't be long' apparently meant 'It will be less than a four-hour wait — hopefully.' So I sat in the large waiting room with around twenty-two other depressed patients for approximately an hour and three quarters, watching intently each time one of them disappeared into a side office, only to be replaced by a new arrival out here in the reception area. Surely my turn would be coming soon.

'Troy?'

'Yup!' I yelped, as I leapt from my seat and darted towards a nerdish-looking man in a white coat.

'Come on in. I'm Dr Harper. So what seems to be the problem today?' he asked.

My response was a little old and over-rehearsed by this point. Not only had I explained my predicament repeatedly in a couple of Sunshine Coast medical centres a month or more before, I'd also been running the story over and over in my head out there in the waiting room. I felt like a criminal about to be questioned by police, but I simply wanted to make sure I gave this man all the information so that maybe I could finally receive a proper diagnosis.

'Well ...' I took a deep, deep breath. 'About a month ago I was on the Sunshine Coast and before that I had just kissed a girl because it was my birthday, but she had a pimple that may not have been a pimple on her upper lip, and then my lips started to tingle, so I went to a doctor who told me my lips were tingling because of a mouthwash infection so he gave me a tablet and I went home, but [*deep breath*] then I started getting a burning feeling on my groin and all around my thighs so I went back to the doctor and had a lot of blood tests but they couldn't find anything wrong with me so I went to another doctor who told me I had prostatitis and gave me tablets and it all went away. [*Sigh.*] But that was a month ago and now it has come back again — the burning, that is — and I'm in pain and pretty freaked out about it ... Could it be a nasty STD? Because I'm a little worried I might've caught a nasty STD.'

The doctor looked at me and nodded. He was very placid for a man who was being ranted at by a terrified stranger. 'Hmmm ...' he hummed, using the universal sound to imply deep thought. 'It would seem that the prostatitis has come back again.'

'Can that happen?'

'Oh sure, it happens all the time. Sometimes you're not on the antibiotics for long enough, so it suppresses the symptoms but doesn't cure the problem. I'll prescribe you a longer series of the antibiotics for now and we'll see how it goes. Oh, and what have you got there?' He had just noticed the sheets of paper I had in my hand.

'These are my test results from a month ago,' I explained. 'I brought them along so you could check them for anything that, um ... they should be checked for.'

I handed the results to Dr Harper, hoping he might discover something the other doctors had overlooked. Poring over the sheets, he suddenly seemed quite concerned and began flicking through the pages for something more. Naturally I panicked.

'Is something wrong?'

'Well, I'm looking for the test results for the prostatitis check. Do you have those?'

'No,' I replied. 'There was no prostatitis check. I was just told I had it. Is that weird?'

'Absolutely! There's a simple urine test that would tell us if you had prostatitis or not, plus the usual check. I can't believe no one ever ran those tests. I'm going to have to do them now if that's okay with you, so we can get a proper diagnosis.'

At that moment all the humour was sucked out of the room. As good as it was to hear the words 'proper diagnosis' at last, his mention of 'the usual check' clouded any joy I might've been feeling. Because every man knows what 'the usual check' means when used in a sentence where the prostate is referenced.

Gulp. Trousers down.

'Lie here on your side and curl up into a ball for me,' he said ominously.

'Uh-huh,' was all I could muster through gritted teeth.

I climbed onto the surgical table and tucked my knees up to my chin, begging for a reprieve like a prisoner in the electric chair praying for that last-minute phone call from the judge. But it wasn't to be.

*Oh!*

'Is that uncomfortable at all?' Dr Harper asked, his lubricated digit probing inside me.

If this had been a social visit then, yes — it would've been extremely uncomfortable. Not only that, but I would've expected some sweet-talk at least, and maybe a meal first, you know?

'Uh,' I said, not really knowing how to answer such an obvious question.

'Fine,' he declared, extracting his finger. 'Put your pants back on and take a seat.'

I let out a sigh of relief and furiously fumbled for my trousers. The sooner they were on, the sooner I could pretend this had never actually happened.

'Well, it's very unlikely that it's prostatitis, because you would've hit the roof with pain if it was. But we'll do some blood and urine tests to confirm and we'll know in two or three days,' he said confidently.

Two or three days. Ah, the waiting game again.

## 7 February — Waiting and burning

You know the drill. (Waiting. Waiting. Freaking out, etc.)

## 8 February — All burning, no waiting

By now the sunburn-like sensation had become so intense that I could barely sit still at work and was sweating a small pool around my chair. So I politely excused myself and ducked back up to the doctor I'd seen two days ago. Even if he didn't have the results yet, I needed to have someone end this pain.

The waiting area was busy as always. Every minute there seemed like a lifetime and every eye seemed to be watching my discomfort with pity. It was horrible. After what felt like an eternity, my name was called, and within seconds I was back in Dr Harper's room.

'Hi again,' he said nervously. 'You look quite uncomfortable there.'

I regaled him with the agonising tale of my increasingly agonising front, and his sudden recollection of my ailment prompted him to check for my results.

'You're lucky. The results came back really quickly. Let's take a look here. Hmm ... uh-huh ... hmmm ... okay ... right ... yep,' he mumbled as he looked over my inner ph balance and nutrient content. 'Yep, just as I thought — no prostatitis. You're in the clear.'

He could tell by the look on my face that this was not the answer I necessarily wanted to hear. 'But you're still in pain, aren't you?' he continued sympathetically.

'Yes. Please can you give me something? *Anything at all*,' I begged, a little over-dramatically.

'I'll give you some painkillers, but that's about all I can do. Sorry. There doesn't seem to be any cause for this at all. Maybe we should wait a few more days and see if it goes away ...'

'Fine,' I answered dejectedly.

Dr Harper handed me a prescription for some sort of painkiller which, I discovered, didn't even need a prescription, as well as a doctor's letter advising that I should take today and the following day off work. I couldn't thank him enough.

I left the useless medical sanctuary and promptly took myself home, to alleviate my suffering with a couple of average-strength painkillers and a looser pair of underpants. But part of me was now internally damaged, mentally at least. For although my Sunshine Coast saviour had given me a confident enough diagnosis and the problem had disappeared for a month afterwards, he was completely wrong in his assessment. After dismissing several possibilities with every passing test, I was now still without any sort of confirmed diagnosis.

Zero diagnosis meant it could've been almost anything that was causing my personal pain, and my mind was awash with fear and a sadness that was tearing me apart. In short, I wasn't in a good place.

# 9 February — Freak-out Friday

In life you can either get busy living or get busy dying. I heard something like that in a film once. Right now, it was high time I got busy sorting this problem out once and for all, even if that meant facing up to some demons I had long avoided.

I awoke on this Friday morning with the pain turned to high and my little man-part hunched and humbled like I'd never seen him before. It was a sorry sight and I wondered if he would ever see the love of a good woman again. All this so soon after his friends down there had received the ultimate accolade, too; 'Testes, 100 per cent' indeed.

Immediately I dressed myself and walked tentatively to the medical centre close to home. Time for a different perspective from a different pair of qualified eyes — and Dr Martyn was the man for the job. I had seen him before for my previously sore bottom and he'd been nothing but direct with me in his assessment of my backside. Perhaps he could do the same for my front.

Barely a moment passed in the waiting room before Dr Martyn, a big bear of a man, beckoned me into his suite and invited me to yet again tell the tormented tale of my sizzling sausage with a side order of hot thighs and the ongoing saga it had created.

He looked at me with disappointment and nodded. 'You probably have herpes,' he said, straight to the point.

'What!?' I yelled. 'Are you sure? I mean ...' I really didn't want to hear this. This was the demon I'd wished to avoid.

'Well, it sounds like herpes. And I can't believe no one has tested you for it yet.'

'But I have no spots! And I didn't even have sex!' I protested. 'And every other doctor has told me it's *not* herpes. How can you be sure when you haven't even looked at it yet?!' I hollered, unbuckling my belt to display the proof.

'I don't need to see it, mate. All the symptoms point to herpes. Sorry.'

He was so matter-of-fact. So blunt. So crippling.

'Either that, or it's hepatitis B,' he finished.

'Really? So it might *not* be herpes?' I asked nervously, at the same time wondering why the hell no one had considered hep B before either.

'Oh, look, nothing is 100 per cent until we do a test, but I can pretty much tell you right now that you've gone and got yourself HSV2. From the sounds of it, she gave you HSV1, which is cold sores, and it's transferred to your groin. Sorry about that, mate.'

Fuck.

The blood tests were painlessly taken as Dr Martyn continued to question me about my previous encounters with doctors and the tests I'd had to endure. 'So none of those idiots ever though to test you for herpes,' he said, rather than asked. 'I can't believe it — how could four doctors miss the mark by so much?'

I didn't reply and he failed to notice the tears welling up in my eyes. Quite simply, I didn't care what he had to say. He'd just told me outright that my worst fear might come true.

'Of course, if it turns out to be all-clear, we'll have to start looking for a cause above the neck,' he added out of the blue.

My ears pricked up. 'Sorry, what did you say?'

'I said, if it's not herpes — which I'm pretty sure it is — then the problem might be up top somewhere.'

'What, like dandruff?'

'Uh, no. Like a mental condition.'

'Oh ... So does that mean I could be mental?'

'We'll have to wait and see,' he concluded with a smile.

In fact, I wasn't really interested in whether or not I was mental. What I'd heard somewhere in this jumbled conversation was that there was still a chance it *wasn't* herpes. That's all I cared about at this point.

'Book in for Monday, first thing, and we'll have the results of these tests for you then, okay?' Dr Martyn told me as we parted company.

I could only hope that Monday would see that small fragment of chance break through and achieve greatness. For now and the weekend ahead, it was back to the waiting game.

## 10–11 February — A plea for divine intervention

More agonising waiting.

Hating life.

Despising my groin.

Stressing.

Praying.

That's right ... I prayed. I hadn't really had many conversations with God, but on this special occasion I literally dropped to my knees and spoke, out loud, to the man upstairs.

'Hi God. Look, I know I can't make deals with you and I know I'm probably not the best, um, believer you've ever had. Sorry about that. But I really need your help right now. If there's any chance you could not give me herpes this time, I would be extremely grateful. I ... I don't know — I'm begging here, God. Whatever it takes. Please, help me out ... Amen.'

That was the best I could manage. A desperate plea disguised as a prayer. I couldn't even remember a psalm to offer or anything, just this pathetic grovelling that would've put a mangy dog to shame.

Looking back now, I'd like to put this in writing: God — I'm sorry. That was terrible. I'll try harder next time, I promise.

## 12 February — D-Day

Having been practically assured that I had either herpes or one of the alphabet of hepatitis infections, I was less than excited about the prospect of meeting with Dr Martyn again. As usual, I was sweating profusely as I made my way into his office for my final judgment.

He looked at me blankly. 'And how can I help you today?' he enquired.

At first I was a little offended. I had assumed that my predicament would've consumed his entire weekend as much as it had mine, but of course in reality he'd seen countless people since our last encounter. My pain was nothing more than a brief moment in his busy working day and, besides, he'd had the entire weekend to unwind afterwards. I felt so alone.

'I was in here on Friday,' I started, trying to jog his memory. 'You did a test for—'

'Herpes!' he yelled excitedly. 'Yes, of course. Let's take a look here. Hmm …'

The pause was gigantic.

'Hmmm …'

He was flicking buttons on his computer, but I couldn't tell if his 'hmmm's were an assessment of my results or him reacting to the adjustments he was making to the monitor's brightness.

'Hmmm …' he said again, still flicking away.

I wanted to punch him.

'Yeah, it seems that nothing has come through yet. They usually take a little longer when the results are positive, because they have to validate them. Sorry about that. I can call you later when they do come through if you'd like?'

'Fuck, yes!' I said quickly, before apologising and stumbling to my feet.

Dr Martyn ushered me out the door without much hesitation and I headed off to my place of work, still in agonising pain and no wiser about my condition. It was a nightmare.

As the day rolled on and the pain tormented my mind and my pants, I felt sick to my stomach every time a telephone rang near my desk. I desperately wanted to know the results — but I really didn't want to know if it meant I had herpes. It was gut-wrenching.

By 3pm I had heard nothing and was beside myself with frustration. I picked up the phone and rang Dr Martyn's office, determined to get the answer I simply had to hear.

Ringing.

'Allo.'

'Hello. My name is Troy Harvey. I was in your office earlier today to get some results from Dr Martyn but he didn't have them, so he was going to ring them through to me. Do you know if he has them yet?'

'I am to be doing the looking for ya reeesults, yes?' the female voice asked in a strong Swedish accent.

'What?'

'Yes, there are not being the reeesults here that you are wanting?' came her response, more confusing that before.

'No. What? I mean, I need to get my results over the phone from Dr Martyn. Do you know if he has them?'

'Dr Martiine does not be giving the reeesults over the tallaphone, no.'

'But ... but he said he would. He said he'd call me.'

'No, you have to be coming in to see him, yes? When would you be coming in to be seeing Dr Martiine?'

'I ... well, first thing tomorrow then, I guess.'

'No, not tomorrow. He is een on the next day only.'

Two more days' wait? Fuck. 'Um ... fine,' I replied, even though it was far from fine. 'Wednesday. First thing. I'll be there.'

'Yes, Mr Harveee, yes. Gud day.'

And with that she was gone and my heart had sunk back into my shoes. It was almost worse than hearing the result itself. Two more days of waiting would be like a month to me. Surely something could be done to fix this injustice — after all, *the man had said he'd call*.

More hours passed and with every tick of the office clock I became more panicked and more frustrated. I would never last another two days. I simply had to try again.

So at 6pm I dialled the number and was relieved when a different voice answered the phone. 'Hello, Dr Martyn's office,' announced a woman in perfect English.

'Hello! Ah, yes! Ah ... um ... My name is Troy Harvey and I was in there today, and Dr Martyn said he would call me later with some test results but he hasn't done so yet. Do you know if he has those results yet? It's pretty *URGENT*!' I blurted.

That last word was emphasised like no word I had ever emphasised before. I don't know that the voice on the other end of the phone even cared all that much, but to me this was possibly the most important call I'd made in a very long time.

'Okay,' she replied. 'He's in with a patient right now, but the moment he comes out I'll get him to call you, all right?'

'Great!' I cried and repeated my phone number in case all their files had been mysteriously destroyed during the course of the day.

After hanging up, I climbed into my car and began the short drive home. The radio volume was set to almost zero and my mobile phone's was moved up to the loudest possible setting, to ensure I wouldn't miss Dr Martyn's life-changing call. I had just crossed Sydney Harbour Bridge when it rang.

*Ring, ring.*

I almost swerved into oncoming traffic.

*Ring, ring.*

I took the first exit off the freeway, pulled into a stranger's driveway and lunged at the phone to take the call. 'Hello!' I screamed.

'Hello, Troy? I have Dr Martyn for you ... One moment,' came the calm voice of the receptionist.

After the briefest of pauses, another, more familiar voice boomed out at me. 'Hello, Troy! How are you?'

'I'm ... er ... Well, I guess I know what you're going to say, so I'm not doing so great, really,' I said dejectedly.

'Well, there's some good news.'

*You ... are ... FUCKING ... kidding me.*

'The tests were all negative,' he continued. 'There's no herpes or hepatitis. There's nothing actually. So maybe we need to—'

*Click.*

I had hung up on the guy before he could squeeze out another word. I simply didn't care. I was in a state of euphoria and ready to climb out of my car and dance among the speeding traffic heading to and from the bridge.

The sun seemed brighter. The harbour seemed more radiant. The cars around me seemed cleaner and the air I was breathing through my open window was suddenly sweeter than ever.

I looked up to the heavens and said a very loud 'Thank you!' before rolling up my window and bursting into tears. Not held-back, manly tears either — but snotty, daggy, *sobbing* tears for a few moments.

Not cool ... but by now I was mentally fucked. This combination of relief and despair was too much for my body to handle. I shook and poured sweat out of every orifice until I'd regained my composure and managed to restart the car and take myself home.

Once inside, I stripped off, climbed into bed, pulled up the sheets and fell asleep almost instantly. It was 7 o'clock in the evening.

## 13 February — Lucky 13th

Waking up after one of the heaviest sleeps I'd had in a long time brought a notable level of contentment. The burning in my groin and surrounding thigh region had reduced dramatically. What was once 100 per cent on fire was now a mere 5 per cent of its strength.

Better still, my mind was clearer — less clouded with dark possibilities, certainly — even though I was still yet to discover the cause of my problem. For, having eliminated the most horrific possible outcomes, only minor ailments remained on my list of likely candidates. So far, I had crossed off the following: herpes, hepatitis (A to Z), gonorrhoea, thrush, chlamydia, HIV, warts, prostatitis, blood pressure, high sugar levels, heat rash, syphilis, urinary tract infection, kidney stones, kidney failure … not to mention explosive groin, smoking wang syndrome and several others I'd basically made up.

And with the burning now less than it had been for the past week or so, and my mind more at ease than ever before, there suddenly didn't seem much to be worried about. Maybe I simply had a sensitive penis that burned whenever someone was talking about it. Maybe I simply needed to get lucky a little more often. Maybe, just maybe, if I ignored the problem now, it would go away completely.

Yeah, right — and maybe one day I'll become the King of England.

# 12
# THE BURNING
# ADJOURNING
## (OR: SO WE KNOW WHAT IT ISN'T —
## BUT WHAT IS IT?)

It was early March, a few weeks since the welcome announcement from Dr Martyn, and in that time my burning had subsided to nothing more than a slight twinge. A 'singe', perhaps. However, as there was still something not quite right about my most prided parts, I remained determined to discover the cause of the problem. By finding the cause, perhaps I'd be able to avoid the problem again in the future. If it was curable, I wanted to cure it; if not, at least alleviate it. And if nothing else, I wanted to give the damned thing a name.

I had made an appointment to see Dr Martyn once more and undertake whatever tests or examinations might've been necessary to finally get to the bottom of the mystery. As it was highly unlikely now that my condition was anything life-threatening, I viewed the ordeal as a sort of medical adventure of discovery. Perhaps people would one day write articles in medical journals about my crotch. I think I'd like that. If I was to be remembered in this world for something, I'd be quite happy if it was for my penis. What man wouldn't?

Filled with a fiery determination that matched the condition in my pants the month before, I marched into the medical centre's waiting area and stormed up to the front desk.

'Can I help you?' a young woman spoke.

I was captivated. The receptionist was unlike any woman I had seen before. Her welcoming features, her eyes like deep blue lakes, and her hair like the romantic swaying reeds that surround the water's edge — she was truly delightful.

'I'm sorry ... I ... uh ... And you are?' I fumbled.

'Marina.'

Of course she was.

'Your name?' she asked, unimpressed by my drooling.

'Oh ... Troy Harvey. I'm here to see Dr Martyn. I have an appointment.'

I was hoping that the last part of my statement would impress her even slightly, since the medical centre featured a large, unmissable sign at the front desk that announced the order of preference for patients in the waiting room: PATIENTS WITH APPOINTMENTS WILL BE GIVEN PRIORITY OVER AND ABOVE WALK-INS OR OTHERS. For the life of me, I couldn't work out who would fall into the category of 'others', but whatever their condition, I was currently at the top of the list.

'Take a seat, Mr Harvey,' Marina said, not even looking up from her computer.

There was nothing I could do but go and sit down, as instructed, among the random walk-ins and creepy 'others' who were occupying the waiting area. My heart was broken.

What else could I do? She probably already knew what I was here for, and most likely wasn't too turned on by the thought of dating a man with a medical problem that resembled the title of a Jerry Lee Lewis song.

I stared at her longingly from my chair. She never looked up. Not once.

'Troy Harvey?' came the all-too-familiar voice of Dr Martyn, who had wandered into the waiting room, oddly undetected for a loud, heavy man. He was looking around quizzically to see which of the six patients before him would be the one to accept his invitation. Personally, after all we'd been through, I was less than happy that he didn't remember me.

'Yup!' I yelped, lunging forwards from my chair with a little too much enthusiasm. This movement was followed by a small stumble and a quick twist of the ankle, which, fortunately, twisted back into its rightful position before causing too much physical damage.

The mental damage — well, that's another story altogether. Not only did I look like a complete schmuck, but five other patients and, sadly, my beautiful Marina, had witnessed my inability to walk like a normal human being. She smirked to herself and tried to suppress a loud laugh, which came out of her nose as a snort instead, thus crushing my ego entirely with one, final blow.

Dropping my head in shame, I wandered past Dr Martyn and into the sanctuary of his private office down the hall.

'You okay?' asked the good doctor, gesturing to my ankle with his eyes.

'Yeah. Fine,' I replied solemnly.

'Good. Good. So what can I do for you today?' Once again, it was as though we'd never met before.

'Well, I had this burning in my groin for a while and—'

'Oh yes!' he exclaimed, suddenly recalling my face or perhaps my crotch. 'That's right — the herpes. Did we ever get the results for that test?'

Did we ever! 'Yeah, it was all negative apparently — or so you told me.' I was starting to regret my decision to come here today. What if, through some miracle of life, he decided to overturn the ruling? Could that happen?

'Oh, that's right. All clear,' he agreed, mostly taking his cues from me. 'You don't even have the cold sore virus in your system, which is amazing since millions of people do. From memory, there was absolutely nothing wrong with your tests. You're perfectly healthy in every way. So what's the problem?'

This question baffled me somewhat because surely he of all people should've known the answer. I mean, he had given me an all-clear for my previous tests, but that still hadn't provided me with a cure for my problem. All it gave me was a couple more ailments to cross off the list of possibilities.

'Um … well, it still hurts. Not the burning as it was, but it's still definitely not right. Something is still, er, *smouldering*,' I offered.

'Well …' He thought for a moment before continuing. 'It seems we have something of an enigma on our hands.'

'Not so much on my *hands*,' I replied, gesturing downstairs.

Dr Martyn was not amused. 'I see,' he said sternly, only to then change his tone completely. 'You know, you may have something that hasn't been discovered yet!'

'Can we name it after me?' I asked eagerly.

'What would you call it?'

'Oh … um … the Troy Harvey Experience,' I announced.

He looked disappointed. Perhaps it was a little too '70s funk for a medical condition.

'No, wait …' My mind was suddenly racing. 'Troy Harvey's Fire Down Below! Troy's Fire Crotch! No, no — the Roasted Nuts of Troy Harvey. I'd love for doctors to have to tell patients they have the Roasted Nuts of Troy Harvey!'

Dr Martyn still wasn't impressed. 'I think we should get

back to finding out what's actually causing the problem before we start on that sort of thing,' he commented, instantly sucking all the fun back out of the room.

'Fine. So what do you think it is?'

'Well, to be honest ...' He was stalling. 'I kind of think it might be ... nothing.'

You could've heard a pin drop.

'Nothing? *Nothing?!* My manhood and thighs had spent much of the last three months feeling like they were submerged in a deep fryer, and you're trying to tell me there's nothing wrong with me?' I was pretty fed up.

'Well ...'

'Look,' I went on, 'it isn't *nothing*. Believe me, it is *something*. I'm not making it up. It genuinely hurts down there. I wouldn't be here if it didn't!'

'I realise that, Troy,' he replied, trying to defuse the mental time bomb. 'I'm not saying that you're not experiencing pain or a burning sensation. What I'm trying to tell you is that you may have simply *created* the problem.'

'What, so I made it up?' I was outraged at such a suggestion.

'Well ... yeah.'

He was noticeably nervous. I was sitting a few inches from him, clenching my fists and steadily changing colour to a possible Hulk-like green. He had every reason to tread carefully.

'You see, Troy, by stressing about your lips all those months ago, you may have transferred the pain to your groin — subconsciously, of course.'

'Can I do that?' I asked, slightly surprised.

'Well, it is possible.'

'But why? Why would my body do that?'

'Stress. You'd be surprised what stress can do to your body. It can manifest itself in some amazing ways. For you, it might've resulted in this burning groin condition because you thought you might have an STD. It's all in your head, is what I'm saying.'

'I'm mental?'

'Not completely,' he replied, half laughing as he did.

'Okay, let's say for a second that this did actually happen,' I began, about to slog him with a doozy of a question and shatter all his theories in one fell swoop. 'But how do you explain the second time, over a month later, when it all came back again? I didn't have sore lips then, so why would I get a burning crotch? What was I transferring that time?'

Nailed it.

'Well, when I say your condition is *made up*, that doesn't mean it doesn't actually exist.'

Very clever, sir. Baffle me with bullshit.

'Troy, your body created a condition from stress, which manifested in your groin. It went away when you stopped stressing about having an STD and forgot about it, right?'

'Right.'

'So, next time you were stressed about something — anything — your body simply chose to reactivate your burning condition again. You have actually *given yourself* a medical condition.'

'You're fucking kidding me!' I blurted out inappropriately.

'Think about it. You told me yourself that the day your tests proved conclusively that you didn't have herpes, or any other STD, the burning lessened considerably. Your *stress levels* dropped, Troy. You have to learn to control them; simple as that.'

'Holy shit,' I continued on my swearing binge. 'So this entire time, my burning bits were only burning because my brain decided to make them hurt. That's pretty fucked up!'

'Not really,' he said. 'Everyone reacts differently to stress. Some people get ulcers or their hair falls out. Personally, I think people can actually give themselves cancer purely by worrying about it. The human body is an amazing thing.'

'And my stress manifests itself in my pants — is that what you're telling me?'

'Not necessarily. You may never experience it again. Next time it might be something else ... somewhere else. Somewhere even worse! So learn to relax a little bit, okay?'

'Well, that's easy for you to say. You don't have great balls of fire!'

'And neither do you. You just think you do.'

'No, no ... I really do. I can feel them,' I insisted.

'I'm sure you can. So stop thinking about them. All your tests say that you're *completely* healthy — you shouldn't even be in here! If you stopped worrying all the time, then there's a good chance I'd never have to see you again.'

'Am I that bad?'

'Not at all. But I'd rather deal with genuinely sick people, if that's okay with you. I feel bad about taking your money,' he added with a chuckle.

'I could always not pay,' I replied with complete sincerity.

'Fat chance. Now go home and relax. You're fine.'

'Are you *sure*?' I challenged one last time, still surprised that my condition was completely made up by my subconscious.

'I am *sure*!' Dr Martyn concluded, guiding me back out to the loving eyes of the wonderful Marina.

'Everything okay?' she asked, perfectly.

'Um ... yeah,' I managed, surprised at both my response and the fact that I was capable of speech in front of someone so captivating.

'Do you want me to send you your bill, or do you want to pay it today?' she continued, wonderfully.

'Uh ... sure,' I answered, suddenly realising I hadn't actually answered her question at all. 'Oh ... I mean, you can send it to me, thanks.'

Promptly, she double-checked my address details and bade me a warm, huggable farewell.

'See ya,' I replied, struggling with the glass exit door. It clearly said PULL. I was suddenly one of those people who pushes a pull-door and causes an embarrassing scene.

'Oh, you need to pull it,' she informed me after the moment had passed.

'I ... er ... uh,' I charmingly replied before stumbling out into the street and out of Marina's life forever. Damn it. Well, she probably had a muscular boyfriend anyway.

I wandered home in something of a daze as the diagnosis set in and I came to the realisation that my brain clearly didn't like me. In my 6-foot-3 body, I seemed to have an incredible amount of internal organs that didn't feel like playing nicely with each other. I wondered if a transplant might introduce a more affable element.

On reaching my couch, I lay down in front of the television, determined to de-stress my body. If my mind had the ability to start this fiasco, it must also have the ability to bring it to an end.

Dozing off in front of *The Simpsons*, I assured myself that all was right with my world. Every test I'd undergone had come back negative and everything in my life could not have been better.

Then, opening my eyes briefly to catch one of the many great sight gags on my favourite TV show, I noticed that my right eye seemed a little blurry to look through. But I figured that was simply due to my highly relaxed state.

At least, I hoped it was. I mean, I wasn't going blind, was I?

*No, no ... Relax. Everything's going to be fine.*

# 13
# THERE'S an OPTOMETRIST IN MY EYE!

'You know he's gay, don't you?' offered up the girl I was dating at the time, as I recounted the harrowing story of what had just occurred during lunch.

'Oh, that's comforting,' I replied sarcastically down the telephone.

'He probably fancied you!' She was almost beside herself with laughter.

'He did *not* fancy me!' I announced loudly enough to inform everybody in the general vicinity. 'He was just ... on top of me.'

This was the second time I'd called her today, and the conversation wasn't going well. In fact, the whole day had gone badly from the moment I'd woken up. So this unsatisfactory phone call wasn't really coming as any great surprise.

Over the past fortnight I had noticed that my eyesight had been rapidly deteriorating. I'd had to wear glasses for years as a result of the genetic deformity my parents had kindly passed on as an heirloom, for me to then pass on to my own children one day if they're lucky. I was familiar with the limitations of my eyes and their inability to make out anything clearly beyond about 10 metres away. It was one of those things you simply learned to accept once you'd seen the price of laser surgery laid out in front of you in a six-point payment plan.

But what had been giving me concern over the past two weeks was discovering that my vision was slightly blurred even if my spectacles were clean and in their rightful place. In fact, on the morning in question, my right eye had seemed to be so blurry, I thought I was staring through Vaseline. And so, through sheer fear of going blind in less than twenty-four hours, I had frantically phoned up my girlfriend at 9am and asked her what I should do.

Now, don't go thinking that I'm the sort of pathetic wimp who goes sulking off to a girl at the first sign of injury or illness … All right, so I generally do — but this time I had a legitimate excuse. My girlfriend happened to work as a receptionist for an optometrist. Therefore, it seemed perfectly rational to think she'd know what the problem was and be able to advise me accordingly.

'I have no idea what would cause that,' she told me that morning, immediately ruining my theory. 'You should probably come in and see Mitch, the optometrist. Can you stop by today?'

'If I can find my way there with one eye, I will,' I'd replied, rather over-dramatising my condition.

'Good. I'll book you in for 1pm. You can come during your lunchbreak.'

I hate going places in my lunchbreak. Not only does the activity in question always take longer than the single hour allowed by my employer, but you also never get to eat lunch. I'd be both blind and starving by the end of this day, not to mention stressed and possibly in a relationship with a man. But we'll get to that soon.

All morning my boss was on my back about some sort of report or document I was yet to produce, and he clearly didn't care much for my excuse that it was difficult to create something without any vision. (I was referring to him, by the way.) By the time my lunch hour arrived, I had fashioned a mock white cane using items I'd found around the office and a shitload of Liquid Paper. Naturally, no one else found it amusing.

I quickly discarded my plans to make a papier-mâché guide dog and headed for the optometrist's. Oddly enough, on arriving there I discovered that my girlfriend was already out to lunch and running some errands. I found it a bit strange that she wouldn't wait around to see her own boyfriend, but you never know what's going through a woman's mind.

I was soon introduced to Mitch by the lunchtime receptionist and led into a small room, which featured a large, mechanical chair and very little else. Mitch immediately re-introduced himself after closing the door behind him and began to enquire about my current condition. He seemed like a nice enough guy, tall with a full head of hair and probably quite handsome, if you're into that sort of thing.

I described my deteriorating vision in great detail, as if trying to convince him that I wasn't mad or simply the hypochondriac partner of one of his employees. I don't know why I went to so much effort; it's not like I was trying to impress him or anything.

'Well, let me take a look and we'll see what's going on here, shall we?' he said, as though this could merely have been a social visit should I not wish to go through with the tests.

'Sure,' I agreed.

'Okay. I'll ask you to stare at the wall in front of you and just relax for me, if you wouldn't mind, Troy.'

Just relax ... Hey, I'd heard that line from medical professionals a thousand times already. He wasn't going to give me a prostate check, was he? That seemed like a very long route to take for an eye check-up.

But before I could blink or leap out of my seat, Mitch was suddenly up in my face like we were slow dancing on a moonlit pier with nothing but the music to guide us. I kid you not — this guy had his cheek firmly pressed against mine as he stared through a tiny metallic instrument and shone an extremely bright light into my eye. I laughed. Nervously.

'Is everything okay?' he asked, as if it was completely normal for us to be snuggling in a back room during lunch.

'Um ... yeah ... I just think it's funny that the light in my eye is so strong and yet you want me to keep it open.' It was a horrible, utterly feeble attempt to make this moment seem less hazardous.

'Yeah, sorry about that,' Mitch replied. 'Not too much longer now. Keep staring straight ahead for me, okay?'

'Sure,' I responded through tight lips.

'Now the other side, please, Troy.' As he gave me this last instruction, he pulled back for a few relieving seconds — only to then throw his leg over mine and press his face up against my other cheek. Yes, people, the man had mounted me!

Looking that closely at my eyes, he must've noticed the shock and horror they were conveying at this point in time. 'Keep staring,' he said, in an apparent attempt to hypnotise me. Possibly.

'Uh-huh,' I managed to mutter before he finally dismounted and stepped a more comfortable distance away from me. *No hug?* I was tempted to say, but sensibly thought better of it.

'So it looks like you're losing some sight in your right eye especially, but the left one is dropping off a bit as well,' he announced casually.

'That doesn't sound good.'

'Well, no. To be honest, it looks like it might be stress-related. Do you get stressed very often, Troy?'

Only when strange men suddenly mount me in a darkened room and give me butterfly kisses ... 'No, not really,' I lied. 'Well, sometimes, I guess.'

'Well, whatever it is, it's only going to get worse,' he told me without a shadow of concern.

'How much worse?' I shot back with great alarm.

'Honestly, I would suggest you could actually lose all your sight at some stage.'

'Blind!' I suddenly felt bad about mocking the visually impaired for most of the morning, back at the office. Karma was clearly about to catch up with me and kick me in the eye sockets.

'Certainly. Within the next few months it could get pretty bad if you don't try to relax.' He delivered this announcement as though he thought it would help lower my heart rate.

'I ... I can't believe it,' I replied, mostly to myself.

It was a horrible moment. There was nothing but silence in the room as Mitch wrote on a tiny notepad and slipped something into my file. It was only when he'd finished and turned back towards me that he saw the look of dismay across my face.

'It's okay,' he said, still obviously not grasping the seriousness of the situation.

'I'm about to go blind! How can that be *okay*?' I yelled back.

'Well, it'll only be temporary ... I did mention that, didn't I?'

Er ... how about *no*! Mitch had neglected to inform me that my rapidly depleting eyesight would only reach rock-bottom for about an hour one day, possibly as I slept, before bouncing back to its normal level of incompetence.

'Ha ha!' he laughed. 'You didn't think it was going to be permanent, did you?'

Perhaps he hadn't noticed my lack of medical qualifications when I'd entered the room. I think he must've been too lost in my eyes.

'Well, I wasn't … sure.'

'No, no — it's all good. You'll be fine. You just have to learn to stress less,' he said finally.

Wow, great advice there, doc. Perhaps you should learn not to tell patients they're about to go blind when you want them to stay calm. Oh, and next time, buy me a drink before we get that close!

My girlfriend was still laughing when I finished recounting the story over the phone. 'He told me you were very handsome,' she said between giggles. 'All the girls here thought you were very handsome too.'

Yeah, because usually people would walk up to a woman and tell her how horrendously ugly her boyfriend is, right? I'm sure they were only being polite.

'But he said you need to relax, darling.' She was now speaking in that tone that makes you feel like a six-year-old.

'I'll do my best,' I replied before hanging up. I wanted to make sure I could find the off button before my sight suddenly disappeared without warning.

As it transpired, my vision never did black out completely. In fact, it improved rapidly, pretty much straight after that one appointment with Mitch the cuddle-bear. The only stress I had now was from trying to explain to my colleagues where I got that stubble rash from.

My boss is still wondering exactly what it is I get up to in my lunchbreaks.

# 14
# WEAK AT THE KNEES

Strange to say perhaps, but when a man damages his leg while running or playing sport, it's a case of the louder the crack, the better. Of course, he doesn't actually want the serious injury that might accompany such an attention-grabbing moment; he'd simply prefer any sport or exercise-related mishap to appear as dramatic as possible. More of a bang than a whimper.

Why? Because it instantly gains him a whopping amount of sympathy from any cute women standing nearby. That's just fact.

Annoyingly for me, my knee gave out one day with no warning and absolutely no noise or dramatic effect that might've helped secure me a wonderful new girlfriend from among any females in the vicinity at the time. No, I was merely conducting a light jog along a path I had lightly jogged so many times before, and a simple, dull ache crept up on me with minimal fanfare but maximum impact.

I tried to proceed along the path but the pain in my knee was getting worse with every step. Eventually I had to pack it in and hobble home. On arriving back at my apartment, after a slow walk that seemed to take forever, I slapped on some Deep Heat cream that had been in a bathroom cabinet for an unimaginable length of time. Then, as a man does in moments of medical emergency, I kicked back on my couch in front of the TV and tried to ignore the pain.

Five days later, as I hobbled around my workplace, loudly moaning about my painful knee condition, a considerate female colleague asked me how I'd managed to do such excruciating damage to myself.

'Oh, I was out running,' I replied, with the usual arrogance we men muster when attempting to impress women with our level of fitness.

'And what happened — did you fall over?'

'No!' I said in mock disgust. 'I ... I don't know. I just hurt it.' It was at this point I realised that, even after nearly a week, I hadn't yet concocted a glorious story of heroism to back up my macho sports injury.

'Well, it looks pretty painful. You should probably go and see a doctor,' she suggested, inadvertently adding herself to the list of women around whom I would never again discuss my ailments.

'Oh ... okay.' I responded, sounding like a pathetic schoolboy who'd just been told to wash up before dinner.

I hate how easily I get talked into doing these things. It almost seems as if a part of me *wants* to see a doctor but simply can't until I'm told to go. It's a male stubbornness that I assume I was born with. Perhaps the Y chromosome stands for 'You-idiot'.

So off I limped, to see a random doctor about another random condition that my body had seen fit to bestow on me. If I were a paranoid man I might think my body is actually trying to destroy me from the inside. I might keep an eye on that theory.

Every step forward seemed to throw me deeper into agony until at last I reached the local doctor's office, around the corner from work, to whinge about my current affliction. For those with a keen eye, you'll have noted that I went to the doctor *around the corner* this time, rather than the medical centre up the road. No particular reason — as you know, I simply like to share my problems around sometimes. Plus, nobody up at the medical centre had managed to cure any of my ailments as yet, so why would I be putting my faith in them now?

Dr Penfold was the charming individual who tended to my throbbing leg that day. After a gentle prod and a push, he announced without a shadow of a doubt that I was suffering from what he termed 'movie-goer's knee'.

'But I don't go to that many movies,' I told him.

'Oh, that's just the name. It refers to people who have some sort of damage immediately below the knee, usually resulting from a lot of standing up and sitting down. Like when you're in the cinema.'

'Movie-goers don't really stand up a lot, though, do they? I mean, they do a lot more sitting than standing, unless it's a Simon Says movie or something ...'

'No, no, Troy — it's only a name. It's not really important. The issue here is that you'll probably need to have an MRI on your leg.'

'What? A brain scan?' I asked honestly.

'An MRI isn't exclusively for your head, it can be for any part of your body. It's a really powerful x-ray that can see in greater detail than a regular x-ray.'

'So why are there still x-ray machines if they've been superseded?' I put to him, hoping a pointless distraction might make him forget to send me for what sounded like a very expensive procedure.

'Well, because the MRI machines are incredibly rare. They cost an absolute fortune. Hence the fees you'll have to pay when you go, I'm afraid.'

Damn it!

'You might also want to contact your knee surgeon, in case,' Dr Penfold threw in casually. 'Who is your regular knee surgeon, by the way?'

My what? *Regular* knee surgeon — like I had a guy standing by? If I did have someone employed purely for my knee, that would be fairly specific of me, doc. I mean, why stop there when I could have surgeons for every part of my body, sitting by the phone awaiting my call, right?

'I … er … I don't have anyone for my knee,' I replied sheepishly, waking up to the reality of life without a 100-strong, personal medical team.

'Fine. You can go to the MRI clinic in your local area, okay? I'll give you a list of people to call at your own convenience, but you'll need to make it soon. That knee's only going to get worse until you do something about it,' he finished ominously.

He then handed me a list of MRI clinics, none of which could in any way have been considered as situated in my local area. It didn't matter, though. It wasn't like I'd be walking to any of them, with my knee the way it was.

Concerned by Dr Penfold's parting thoughts, I made a booking at the closest MRI clinic on the list and managed to suffer through two more days until the appointment arrived.

Still limping and moaning endlessly about my lot in life, I strode brokenly into the clinic's reception area, where I instantly noticed a ludicrous level of silence for a room filled with people. The staff seemed to be moving about without making a sound, while patients sat forlornly on worn brown couches, staring hopelessly into the distance. It was most foreboding.

Not wishing to disturb the awkward hush, I meekly announced my arrival to the woman behind the front desk. She nodded and smiled like a nervous hostage who'd been told to give nothing away by an armed gunman under the counter. I smiled back, surreptitiously leaning forwards slightly to check that there wasn't a shotgun pressing into her stomach, before moving off to a seat among the zombies. What was everyone so concerned about?

After a short period of staring at the other patients and receiving little to no reaction, I saw a nurse approaching me. 'Are you Mr Harvey?' she asked quietly.

'Yeah!' I exclaimed with far too much enthusiasm for the room. Two people visibly jumped.

'Come with me.'

She then led me down the hallway to a bright room with lockers along the wall. 'It's like being back at school,' I noted out loud.

'Not quite,' she replied in a tone that turned my stomach. 'You'll need to remove your clothes, any jewellery and anything else metallic from your body. You can put them in one of these lockers. Then throw on the gown and come through to the other room, please.'

She was right — I didn't remember school being anything like this. Mind you, it might've been a lot more fun in some ways if it had been.

After stripping down and adorning the ill-fitting gown, I moved into the room next door to behold the frighteningly large MRI machine. It looked exactly like the frighteningly large MRI machines you see in those depressing medical dramas on TV. There was nothing happy about this room at all.

'Now I want you to relax,' the nurse told me.

That word again — while much beloved by medical folk, it always lets you know when something awful is about to happen. I was ready to run and I think the fear showed on my face.

'There's nothing to be afraid of here, Mr Harvey. All you have to do is lie down and relax and it will all be over very shortly.'

'How shortly?' I asked as she dug through drawers for something else to alarm me with.

'It takes about forty-five minutes for the machine to do its job. Now, I'm going to place these earplugs in your ears to protect them from the noise, okay?'

'The *noise?*'

'Yeah. It can get pretty loud sometimes.'

Who ever heard of an x-ray machine getting loud?

'Seriously, just relax,' she repeated, stuffing the plugs into my ears and instantly muffling everything she said from that moment on.

I climbed onto the cold metal slab and stared into the scary tunnel that lay waiting to consume me.

'Are you comfortable?' she asked, barely audible.

'I guess.'

'Good. You'll need to be comfortable, because once we start, you can't move at all. If you move even an inch, we might have to start again. Okay?'

Was she serious? Surely one of the worst things someone can tell you to do is lie completely still for a set amount of time because you immediately become hyper-aware of every part of your body. Every hair on your being itches like it has never itched before. Your toes and fingers feel fake, glued on even. Your breathing is loud and irregular, tormenting your brain as it tries to ensure that no part of your irritated body does anything it shouldn't be doing, for fear of having to undergo the whole procedure again. In short, for me, being instructed not to move a muscle for forty-five minutes was borderline torture.

'I'll be fine,' I bleated. 'Er, but what if I get an itch?'

'I'll be in the next room watching you through the glass. I'll be able to hear everything, so you let me know if there's a problem and I'll come in and rub it for you. Okay?'

It sounded saucy. Except ... sorry, did she just say she'd be in another room *watching me through glass*? 'Um ... is this dangerous?' I asked as she started to leave.

'Mrphhhp sombshhshh,' is all I heard as the earplugs expanded and she ran for her own safety. 'Ar ooh o-aay?'

Her voice appeared to be coming from a million miles away,

but I figured she was either asking if I was okay or telling me to get ready to start. Either way, there was no turning back now.

*Bvvvvvvvvmmmmmmmm* ...

The metal slab I was on drifted towards the tunnel of doom, which eventually enveloped me completely and left me with nothing to stare at but the plain white interior of my metal tomb. If this was as bad as it got, then everything would be okay. Sure, it was pretty dull in there, but as long as nothing el—

*BRRRRRRRRRRR TANK-TANK-TANK-TANK GRRR-GRRR GAT-GAT-GAT NNVVVVVVVVVV TTTTTT-ZZAT.*

Holy fuck!

That sound is, to this day, the angriest sound I have ever heard coming from a machine. It was so ridiculously loud that I feared the earplugs must've shot out of my ears with the sudden shock. It was like a jackhammer with a megaphone attachment. The staccato clicking and clanking was rapid and horrible, and any minute I expected lasers to shoot out of the tunnel walls and burn me to within an inch of my life.

And the brutal noise just kept on coming.

*BRRR GA-DANK GA-DANK GA-DANK TONK-TONK-TONK HARRRR-GRRR VIT-VIT-VIT NNNNNNNNIDDD BA-ZUNK!*

It was furious. Had the machine suddenly transformed itself into a giant Deceptacon and begun destroying everything in its path, I wouldn't have been the least bit surprised.

I now understood why the patients in the waiting room were staring blankly at the walls. They must've experienced this sound before and knew what lay ahead for them today. Why had none of them warned me, though? Not that it would've prepared me if they had. *Nothing* could've prepared me for this violent torment, during which my job was to lie perfectly still and pretend like everything was fine. So far I had been doing wonderfully.

*BUDADBUDABUDABUDA TANK-TANK-TANK-TANK ZAAAA ZAAAA TAT-TAT-TAT WHEZZZZZZZZZZZZZZZ ZUZANK!*

*Hic!*

What the hell was that? Was that the machine? Is it possible that the MRI tunnel was actually devouring me?

*Hiccup!*

Oh fuck. That wasn't the machine at all. It was *me*.

*BRRRRRR KERCHECKZACHECK NEERRRRRRRRRR TAC TAC TAC TAC BAZIIING GADADADADDADDDDD FLINK!*

*Hiccup!*

I *knew* something would go wrong. You can't ask the human body to lie that still for so long without it rebelling. It simply can't be done!

*Hiccup!*

Without warning, the mechanical aggression then seemed to grind to a most welcome halt. Temporarily or for good, I had no idea. 'Is everything all right in there?' my nurse asked loudly through a tinny speaker.

'Uh-huh,' I squeaked back.

*Hiccup!*

'I need you to lie completely still, Mr Harvey. You seem to be moving around a little bit. Are you sure you're okay?'

'Fine!' I replied through gritted teeth, desperately trying to alter my breathing and put an end to this madness.

*DAT DAT DAT DAT BUDUDUDDUDUDUDDUDA PEZZZZZZZZZZZZZ ZINK ZANK Z BAZZZZZINK CRANK CRUNK ZANK!*

She had turned the machine back on within seconds of my response, and the sudden return of ear-shattering noise shocked me all over again. I hoped it would be enough to scare the hiccups out of my system.

*BRRRRRRRRRRRRRRR   DADADADADDADADAD-*
*DADDADADADDADD   PACHENK   PACHINK   PACHONK*
*HNNNNNNN BZZZZZZZZZART!*

Wait for it ... Waiting ... Waiting ...

Nothing! I was sure it had —

*Hiccup!*

Fuck. The last thing I needed was to have to repeat this
entire, god-awful process, if my current fidgeting meant we had
to start again. It seemed like I'd been in here for ten hours by
now, and already I wanted to destroy anything mechanical in my
apartment the moment I got home. I didn't need the reminder.

*BRRRR   TANK-TANK-TANK-TANK   GRRR-GRRR   GAT-*
*GAT-GAT NNVVVVVVVVDD TTZZART!*

*Hiccup!*

Well, the machine seemed to be continuing regardless of my
ongoing air attacks. Perhaps it wasn't as bad as I thought.

'You're still moving around in there, Mr Harvey,' came the
nurse's voice once more, angrier this time. 'Not long to go now.
Please try to lie still, okay?'

*How long is 'not long'?* I thought to myself, fearful of speaking
aloud in case it moved me that terrifying inch she'd spoken of
approximately three days ago.

*Z Z Z Z Z Z Z Z Z Z Z Z A A A A A R R R R R K K K*
*DIDIDIDIDIDIDIDT MUZZZZZZ SHENK SHENK SHENK*
*SHENK PHIZZZZORT!*

*Hiccup!*

Surely people were missing me by now. It felt as though I'd
been lying there for a week, so why had nobody come looking
for me yet? I was a hostage in a metal tube of death — but how
could I get a signal to the outside world?

*BACHINK KERCHUNK MIZZZZZZZZZZZZZUUUUT*
*GAT DAT GAT DAT KUDAKUDAKUDAKUDA GANK!.*

*Hiccup!*

*Dear God, please make it stop* ... The sound had invaded my skull and shattered my brain into a million tiny pieces. Every part of my body felt like it weighed a tonne and was so tense that I feared rigor mortis had officially set in. How much longer could a man endure this kind of attack on his mental state?

*BIZZZZZZZZZZZZZZZ AZUZAZUZAZUZAZU PIKA PIKAPIKAPIKA MUZZZZZZZZZZ DAT GAT DAT GAT KERHUNKEN SPLANK!.*

*Hiccup!*

The racket was getting louder now. I desperately wanted to scream at the top of my lungs and wrestle my way out of this MRI-monster's clutches. I had to. This was more than I could stand. My last straw had been well and truly snapped in several places. If I heard those sounds for one more minute, I was going to break free and run down the hallway (or at least break into an efficient hobble), yelling at all those in the waiting room to get out now, before they too were subjected to this evil torment.

'Mr Harvey?' It was that familiar voice again, coming at me through the tinny speakers. 'You can relax; we're all done now. How are you feeling?'

'Oh ... fine,' I lied. No point in making a scene, after all.

Within seconds the metal slab was drifting slowly out of the horror tunnel, at which point I noticed that my hiccups had completely disappeared. Naturally.

'So that wasn't too bad, was it?' asked my happy little nurse, now back in the room with her hand on my shoulder.

'No, it was fine ... Not a problem.'

My lip was trembling a little but I don't think she noticed. What she might've been aware of, however, was the swiftness with which I left the room, clothed myself and exited the building to once again feel sunlight on my face and taste sweet, sweet freedom.

All up, I had been in there for about forty-two minutes.

* * *

One week later I was asked by Dr Penfold to come in for the results of my ordeal. He took a close look at the scans and informed me that I had a condition known as patella tendonitis — which sounded nothing like the movie-goer's knee he'd assured me I was suffering from last time we spoke.

'And what exactly is nutella takeabitus?' I asked ignorantly.

'*Patella tendonitis* simply means that you have an inflamed tendon just below the front of your knee.'

'Oh. So it's only a sore knee? Sounds a bit pathetic really, considering what I had to go through to find out.' I was actually quite disappointed by this development.

'Well, not really,' said Dr Penfold, offering a glimmer of hope. 'It's extremely painful, in fact, and will require quite a bit of therapy to put right. It's no wonder you can't walk properly.'

I felt justified. Plus, I wouldn't be requiring my knee surgeon, as it turned out, and could possibly release him from my staff.

But there was a bigger upside, as part of Dr Penfold's verdict was absolute music to my ears. To cure my condition, I would have to visit that most hallowed medical professional, the one that men will willingly see, without any prompting from a female in their lives. Yes, I was going to have to visit ... The Physio.

The grinding, clanking, angry aural attack I'd recently endured was now worth the nightmares it had given me since then. Why? Because a physiotherapist's office is the coolest place on earth a guy can get to say he's going to. Quite simply, the physio maketh the man.

Guys love telling people they've been to see their physiotherapist. The physio implies sports-related injury, after all. Now, ask a man to show off his sporting prowess and, no matter how limited it may be, he'll do his best to convince you that he could've played at a professional level with the best of them. But better still, by telling women we visit a physio, we get to bypass any display of this prowess and move straight into the sympathetic clutches that await. (Or so we imagine.)

If a guy has to see a physiotherapist, he will tell *everyone*. 'Just off to the physio for my knee!' you'll hear echoing down every office corridor. Or: 'Got a back thing — gotta go see my physio!' And by telling absolutely everybody, we let them know we're active, sporty, incredibly manly and tragically injured all at the same time.

Men respect other men with physio appointments. Sports stars have physio appointments; ipso facto, regular guys with similar appointments must be sports stars also. It all makes perfect sense, and I couldn't thank Dr Penfold enough.

The thing is, I never actually went to the physio ... Oh sure, my doctor had given me the green light to start announcing to the world that I was in *need* of a physio, but a lack of time and financial stability prevented my dream from ever becoming a reality.

Having phoned the recommended physiotherapists in the area, I was informed that they were only ever open between 11am and 3pm, Monday to Friday. To me, this seemed ludicrous. Didn't they realise that many of us humble human beings *weren't actually sports stars* and therefore had to work during these limited hours? Unbelievable. Add to that the simple fact that every time I left my place of employ to undergo such pricey therapy, I would be docked for the time I was away — meaning that, after a few visits to these glorified gym instructors, I'd be financially ruined, albeit able to walk properly perhaps.

No, it simply wasn't to be. A far easier way to repair my damaged patella, it seemed to me, was to download the required physiotherapy moves on the internet and perform them at home for almost a week — before giving up and merely hoping the knee would repair itself.

Of course, that didn't stop me telling the entire world and anyone else who would listen that I was *doing* physio, you understand ... It was slightly misleading of me, I admit. But it was such a great thing to drop into conversations with beautiful women at parties or in the pub. Their eyes would glaze over and they'd begin to stare around the room without any hint of interest at all, but I knew that deep down they thought I was cool. How could they not? I was doing physio.

And for the past two or three years I have managed to continue this ruse at every function I've attended. Because my knee never actually got better. Okay, it isn't as terrible as it was and I can manage a light jog every once in a while; but my limp is still there on a cold day and the pain still makes me wince if I stand up too quickly, or if I'm asked to kick a footy around with some mates.

I never was very good at sport. I'm better off having an excuse to get out it — and besides, claiming that I'm doing physio puts me on a higher pedestal with work colleagues anyway. Getting better would be a tragedy. So, I'll keep 'doing physio' for as long as I can get away with it.

Ironically, giving myself a sore knee is probably the most impressive sporting achievement of my entire life. I wonder if they make a trophy for that?

# 15
# Laser Eyes

As mentioned previously, my eyesight was always perfect until after high school. I'd love to have been one of those kids who was getting bad grades for years and then suddenly discovered it was because I couldn't see the blackboard properly, but the truth is I was just getting bad grades. Damn it.

Soon after high school ended, my perfect vision began to slip somewhat, until after about a year I could no longer see things in the distance very well. Squinting helped, but I found it difficult to enjoy an entire night's TV viewing this way. Not to mention how unsafe people must have felt when they passed me in traffic.

Something needed to be done.

Eventually I found myself wearing glasses, but only when I really needed to. I hated the way they felt on my face and also the way they'd slip off my nose every time I got sweaty. I also worried that they didn't suit me, but repeated reassurance from family and friends finally got me over my vanity and I continued to wear them for almost ten years.

Regular visits to the optometrist were *usually* uneventful and nothing but an expensive chore (the aforementioned snuggling with Mitch being the only real exception), but in the back of my mind I had always wished for a way out of this ocular impediment that life had handed me.

Then one day it happened.

After breaking a pair of four-hundred dollar 'unbreakable' specs by sitting on them, I made a visit to an optometrist who changed my world forever.

She was a young woman, fairly attractive and extremely keen to fit me with the most expensive pair of frames she could find. At first I enjoyed her playful salesmanship and think she may have even winked at me from the other side of the floor a couple of times. Of course, I can't be sure as she was too far away for me to actually see, but lets assume she did.

Together we worked our way through almost every pair of frames on the shelf, with me trying on each one only to be met with her head shaking 'no'. By the end of the facial fashion parade, she finally said something to me that I really did not want to hear.

'You just don't look good in glasses.'

This hurt. Not only because she was quite pretty herself and had been fairly brutal in her delivery of the line, but also because I had been wearing glasses (in public sometimes!) for almost ten years. Why had everyone lied to me? How could they be so cruel to a 'blind' man?

'You should think about laser surgery,' she continued.

'Lasers, eh?' I said, immediately conjuring up images of green rays shooting from my eyes and destroying evildoers.

'It's pretty safe these days,' she continued, ignoring my head-tilt and the way I was cartoonishly stroking my chin.

I don't really know about that last statement from her. Honestly, how safe can it be to shoot laser beams into your eyes? I don't care if you are a medical professional, the moment you're playing with lasers you start coming across like a mad scientist hell-bent on world domination. Or maybe I watch too many movies.

Regardless, she'd put the thought in my mind now and there was no turning back. I looked like a freak whenever I wore glasses, apparently, and the crow's feet around my eyes from squinting were starting to look more like those of an ostrich.

I quickly purchased the cheapest and, somehow, least flattering pair of glasses the optometrist had on offer and raced home without wearing them to investigate the realities of laser eye surgery.

Here is the first thing most people discover: It costs a fucking fortune.

For a while I figured that fact would also be the last thing I discovered about the procedure since I didn't have the equivalent of a major Lotto win sitting idle in my bank account, but just as I went to give up and squint at the television for a while, I stumbled across a website that read: 'Laser eye surgery — both eyes for only $800. Call now!'

Now, for me $800 is still a lot of money — but nowhere near as impossible to source as the tens of thousands of dollars the other companies were trying to take me for. Surely there must be a catch?

They say that when one of your natural senses becomes weak, your other senses are heightened to compensate for it. I sometimes think that my poor vision led to a heightened sense of imagination, as I was now envisioning a homeless man in an alleyway with one of those laser pointers you use in a business meeting, holding me down while he melted my eyeballs.

This price seemed too good to be true so I immediately picked up the phone to enquire as to why they were so ludicrously affordable. A man answered.

'Welcome to Laser Eyes, how can I help you?'

He didn't sound homeless, but I couldn't really be sure.

'Hi, I, um, I wanted to ask about your laser eye surgery. I wanted to know how come, well, er... Why are you so cheap?'

The man laughed briefly then spoke in a very calming manner.

'We get that question a lot. Our surgeon is a specialist in the field and generally performs around 25 laser operations a day, so he doesn't need to charge the earth like other companies.'

A quick calculation in my brain worked out that surgeon probably makes a shitload of money.

'But is it any different to the more expensive places? I mean, what would I be missing out on?'

'Sir, it's exactly the same as anywhere else. We perform the surgery on a Friday and you rest for the weekend. On the Monday we see you again to check it's all on track, then you have a year's worth of free consultations with us, should you need them.'

'Why would I need them?' I asked nervously.

'Don't worry,' he reassured me, 'most people don't.'

If only he knew that when it comes to medical procedures, I wasn't like *most* people.

'Would you like to come in tomorrow for a free initial consultation to see if you qualify for surgery?' he asked.

'Sure,' I said, still stunned that there seemed to be, so far, no catches at all. Not only that, but he'd already used the word 'free' twice in conversation. I like the word 'free'.

So with that he took down my details and made arrangements for me to bring my eyes in the next day for a thorough, professional inspection.

After hanging up the phone, I immediately attempted some in-depth online research about the company, but was surprised to find very little information about them anywhere. Perhaps they were a new company? Or maybe all of their patients had been left blind and unable to navigate the World Wide Web! No, wait … surely their family and friends would write something about that somewhere. Not to mention news coverage.

It seemed generally odd, and the fact that they could make an appointment for me the very next day made me wonder where these patients for '25 surgeries a day' were coming from. The way he had spoken about the business, it sounded like you couldn't move in their offices for all the patients stumbling about blindly.

I thought about it for a little while longer — longer than any rational person would, actually — before deciding that the best thing to do was to slowly back away from the computer and wait until my visit with Laser Eyes to make my final assessment.

After a night of restless sleep I drove dangerously through the morning traffic, squinting the entire way, mostly using The Force more than my actual eyesight to guide me to my destination.

Upon arrival I discovered that the building I was about to enter was quite modern and welcoming. There were no signs guiding me down a side alley to a homeless man with a laser pointer, as I had half expected, but rather a beautiful glass exterior and large, easy-to-find doors that were almost impossible for even the blindest man to miss. Inside was even more pleasant, with a delightful lounge area, plenty of indoor plants and about five staff members working frantically behind a large desk.

'Welcome!' one of the staff said, smiling at me the moment I stepped inside.

I told them my name and why I was there and within minutes was offered a complimentary coffee and ushered towards the lounge to relax while they prepared the machinery for my eye examinations. It was all surprisingly professional and everyone was nothing short of charming.

Naturally, rather than feeling reassured by all of this, I became more and more sceptical as the minutes ticked by. One of the things I couldn't help but notice immediately after taking my seat was that all five staff members were wearing glasses.

Why in the world would anyone employed at a laser eye clinic still be suffering from a visual affliction? Was there not a staff discount for surgery or did they know something I didn't?

I won't lie, I was a little thrown.

Mind you, I was even more thrown by the display on the wall behind the main counter. It was decorated with almost 20 degrees, diplomas, awards and salutes to the man who, I had been earlier informed, would be conducting my surgery if my eyes were smart enough to pass their initial exams. You'd think this amount of education and accolade would provide me with some increased level of confidence — and normally it would — except for one small discrepancy.

Every single framed document featured a different spelling of the surgeon's name. I kid you not.

One degree read 'Dr Toby Gillen'. Another presented 'Dr Tobi Gillan'. Beneath that one, 'Dr Tobe Gillian'.

Alarm bells were ringing loudly in my tiny brain now as I continued to assess the documents on display. I can understand the occasional typo or misspelling of someone's name, but 20 times on the most important paperwork of an individual's career seemed a little odd to say the least. What was this man hiding? Was he on the run from the law? Could he cure eyesight but not dyslexia?

I was sweating bullets by the time a kindly young woman by the name of Sophie came to take me through the examination process.

I won't waste your time with a detailed description of the tests that were conducted, other than to mention that I passed every one of them with flying colours — which basically meant that I was legally blind enough to warrant having laser beams shot violently into my eyeholes and pay $800 for the privilege.

The one thing Sophie did tell me as I thanked her for her time was that I was fortunate because I had 'amazing tear ducts' and therefore wouldn't suffer from any dryness after the surgery.

Exactly what any man wants to hear: I am genetically designed to be a sook. Brilliant.

Caught up in the euphoria of passing the tests and roundly applauded by the five staff members still working frantically behind the counter, I figured it would be best to ride this high straight into surgery and enquired as to when would be the next available time to potentially melt my eyeballs.

'Friday', I was informed.

'What? *This* Friday ... as in three days from now?' I responded, amazed by the speed at which this was all taking place. 'Uh ... I guess so.'

And with that I was booked, handed two prescriptions for mysterious drugs and told to return on the Friday morning 'relaxed and ready to rest over the weekend'. Little did they know that the word 'relaxed' wasn't really in my repertoire when it comes to medical procedures.

'What are the prescriptions for?' I asked one of the frantic staff members behind the counter.

'One is a powerful painkiller and the other will help you sleep over the weekend while you heal. Oh, and you really should buy a *lot* of eye drops to keep your eyes moist after the surgery.'

'I was told I have amazing tear ducts,' I mentioned proudly. The woman behind the counter smiled.

'Seriously, get some eye drops,' she said matter-of-factly before retuning to her frantic duties, whatever they were. Hopefully it didn't involve responding to legal action.

Apart from the fact that everyone in the place was wearing glasses and the surgeon's real identity was one of the world's greatest unsolved mysteries, the other thing weighing on my mind as I strolled back to my car were the words *powerful painkillers*. Just how powerful did they need to be? What exactly was I about to endure?

As usual, I had to stop for a few moments and reassure myself that I was probably overreacting and that hundreds of thousands of people have had laser eye surgery in the past and never had a problem.

No, everything would be fine come Friday. *Surely*.

The next couple of days were not good ones for me. I much prefer to dive into a situation without thinking too much about the consequences, because once I do begin to analyse the consequences I tend to chicken out and run a mile. Constantly talking myself around to thinking logically and rationally is not really my forte.

So by the time Friday morning rolled around, my stomach felt like a swarm of butterflies caged in a bundle of nerves.

I had purchased the powerful painkillers, sleeping tablets and a small packet of eye drops, just in case my sooky genes didn't kick in when they were supposed to. I was ready for the big laser lightshow.

Returning to the pleasantly decorated venue I had visited earlier in the week, I was surprised to see so many people nervously reclining on the comfortable lounges, while the formerly frantic staff sat calmly behind their counter casually processing the patients' details and telling them in hushed tones to take a seat. Where had all these people come from?

My details were checked and I joined the throng of hopefuls as we sat quietly, trying everything we could to avoid conversation until one by one the numbers dwindled and patients were taken behind closed doors – never to be seen again.

I've seen movies like this. I didn't like them.

Suddenly my name was called and, after looking around to confirm that there weren't any other Troy Harveys standing by for surgery, I swallowed hard and made my way behind the door from which no one ever returned.

Fuck.

Inside the brightly lit room was a large, reclining medical chair, a hulking great machine that I assumed to contain laser technology, and four nurses wearing facemasks, who positioned me on the chair as we awaited the arrival of the variously named doctor.

About 5 minutes later, the door opened and a friendly looking man reached out his hand to shake mine.

'Hi Troy,' he announced, blatantly neglecting to say his own name back, 'I'll be doing your surgery today. There's nothing to worry about. Lie back and we'll be done in about 15 minutes. Try to relax.'

Think now about every horror film you have ever seen. To me, the scariest ones are when everyone is overly friendly, wearing masks and closing in on you with medical equipment. That's what this felt like, especially when I noticed the giant, dead Hunstman spider in the plastic cover of the light directly above me. At least, I assumed it was dead. I hope so. I *hate* spiders.

While I stared at the motionless arachnid above me, Dr Tobias Gilliam began *STICKY TAPING MY EYELIDS BACK*. Seriously. I throw up in my mouth a little every time I think of that moment. Not only because it was even more like a horror film now that ever, but because I had a terrible fear of what might happen when the sticky tape was removed. What if it ripped off my eyelids? Mind you, it could give my eyebrows a bit of a wax, which would be handy.

Breathe, Troy. Breathe.

'Now, I'm just going to put some drops in to numb your eyeballs so you won't feel anything when I strip them back a little,' offered Dr *Tobby Gillane*.

Did he say he was going to strip my eyeballs back? Are you *fucking* serious?

Taking a deep breath to calm myself, I noticed that my hands had gripped the side of the chair I was seated in so hard that I thought I was going to rip through the fabric.

'Just relax,' the doc reminded me as he flooded my eyes with liquid.

I tried to force out a smile but it wasn't happening.

A half a moment later I was experiencing the most horrifying sensation I have ever endured. The man was SANDING MY EYEBALLS!

I know it sounds odd, but it's the only way I can describe what was going on. Dr *Tobey Gilien* was furiously rubbing what appeared to be sandpaper across my eyes while all I could do was stare in horror and feel my toes curl up like the shoes of an elf.

Shouldn't I have been unconscious or something? It was bad enough that I had to *sense* what was taking place, but to be forced to watch it at close range made it infinitely worse. If it continued much longer I was definitely going to paint this man's face with vomit.

I imagine that was what the other four nurses were there for – to restrain patients and clean up their hurl – because so far not one of them had contributed anything to the events of the day other that to watch on with glee. *Those sick bitches.*

The eyeball sanding concluded mere seconds before I was about to reach up and punch the doctor in the face, and for a few moments I was able to compose myself and start breathing again like a normal human being.

That's when the laser machine began to warm up.

It was like someone had switched on a nuclear power grid in a movie from the '80s. Loud, whirring noises filled the room and the light above me that once contained a giant spider dimmed a tiny bit. It also didn't contain a giant spider any more.

Fuck.

Suddenly Dr *Tobay Gillun* leapt out of his chair and swiftly manoeuvred the loud machinery over my face and instructed me to stare at the small, illuminated green dot that was now directly in front of my right eye. My vision was somewhat blurry thanks to a combination of drops, eyeball shavings and my overly active tear ducts, but I managed to stare at that little green dot as though my life depended on it until he told me to stop.

I was sure nothing had happened because I never once saw a laser fire into my face, but upon questioning the surgeon I was assured the necessary activities had occurred. 'Now the other one,' he instructed.

He slid the machine over my left eye and again told me in no uncertain terms to stare directly at the little green light. The only problem was, the little green light had turned red.

'There's only a red light."

'Are you sure? There should be a green one,' he said nervously.

'I swear there's only a little red light. Nothing green at all!'

'Oh well, it *should* be okay,' he replied. 'Stare at the red light then.'

This all seemed a little too blasé to me. The man was holding a nuclear device above my head and about to shoot lasers into my skull, yet even though something was clearly malfunctioning with the equipment, he seemed determined to continue and get through his daily quota of 25 patients.

I was too nervous to argue and stared at the red light until he told me to stop. Then, without any warning, he dropped a pair of contact lenses into my eyes, ripped off the sticky tape (thankfully leaving my eyelids attached) and announced triumphantly that the job was done.

He then removed a rubber glove, politely shook my shaking hand and instructed me to follow one of the nurses out a different door to the one I had walked through originally, into a small dark waiting room, where I sat alone wondering if maybe that spider had found its way into the room as well.

Luckily, I'll never know.

After around 15 minutes of sitting alone in the dark I was joined by a friendly nurse. It was Sophie, who informed me that I needed to take the drugs I had purchased earlier and go home to rest until Monday. 'Oh, and one important thing,' she said sternly, 'Do not remove the contact lenses or even touch your eyes until Monday. Leave them in and get some sleep. On Monday the doctor will remove them and your vision will be greatly improved. We'll see you then.'

I can tell you now, I have no idea how I got home from the surgery. After Sophie guided me out onto the street I became drowsy and nauseous and could well have slept in the gutter until family came to my rescue, I honestly don't know.

What I do remember is waking up sometime on Saturday night and rubbing my itchy left eye furiously until it dawned on me what I was doing.

I stopped immediately and opened my eyes, waiting for some sort of vision to come. My right eye slowly adjusted to the room and could see almost perfectly even though it was dark, but the left one was blurred beyond belief. What had I done? Did I lose the contact lens? How could I tell if it was still in there?

I began to search the bed frantically, looking for a tiny piece of clear plastic that would have been hard enough to find in full light with 20/20 vision, let alone with half-decent vision in one eye on poorly lit, dark bed sheets.

It wasn't to be. The contact lens was nowhere to be found, as far as my limited finding abilities could determine, so I simply lay there in a sweat trying to focus my left eye on anything I could until I drifted off to sleep again and forgot for a while my impending life of sight through one eye.

I must say, whatever those tablets were that powerfully prevented pain and made me sleep well were certainly working. I never felt a thing and only woke two or three times before early Monday when it was time to face the music with the surgeon, whom I now realised had never even revealed his face to me, let alone his identity.

Frighteningly, my left eye was still unimproved. While my right eye was seeing the world in a whole new light, my left made everything look like it was being observed through soup. I was terrified.

Back at the surgery for my third and, *apparently*, final visit, I was led into a room full of all-new equipment and machinery and told to wait for Dr *Toaby Gillene* to arrive. I found it extraordinary that the first time I might actually see the man's face unmasked would be on a day that one of my eyes simply wasn't functioning. Maybe I'd only see half his face and keep the mystery alive forever?

Seconds later the doctor entered the room and he looked ... like a regular guy. Nothing exciting or alarming. He bore no resemblance to any prominent international figure using noms de plume or masks to keep their identity concealed, much to my overactive imagination's disappointment.

He reached out and shook my hand with a smile then asked me how things were going with my eyes.

'Well ...' I began, taking a deep breath, '... I kind of woke up on the weekend and I was drowsy and I forgot where I was or what had happened and didn't realise I was rubbing my left eye for a while until I remembered that I wasn't meant to be rubbing my left eye and think I might have ruined the surgery and lost the contact lens because now I can't see anything and might be blind for life.'

'Riiiiight,' he replied. 'Let's take a look, shall we?'

I hastily threw myself behind a machine in the belief that the sooner my eyes were looked at, the less permanent damage would be done to the slowly dying left one. The doctor moved in for a closer look.

'Well, the contact lens is still in there,' he said.

I sighed a deep sigh.

'But you've pushed it behind your eye somehow,' he concluded.

I almost threw up a little.

'I can see a tiny bit of it sticking out the corner of your eye, so I'm going to have to pull that out with tweezers. Please sit very still for a moment.'

'Are you saying the contact lens is ... *TOUCHING MY BRAIN*?' I screamed, gagging slightly at the same time.

'Just relax, Troy,' he replied, never actually answering my question.

As he gripped the tiny lens with the tweezers, I felt it squish along the side of my eyeball and possibly nudge the part of my brain that once housed information about trigonometry. Well, that's gone now.

Having the contact lens out didn't improve the vision from my left eye, though, so I was still extremely concerned, as well as slightly nauseous from the whole lens on the brain incident.

'Let me take a closer look at your eyes through this scope,' he insisted, pushing yet another piece of equipment in front of my face and peering through the other side of it.

'Well, your right eye is great. That really looks good. Your vision on your right will get even better over the next few weeks, so that's really great.' As he told me this I couldn't help but feel he was doing more to congratulate himself on his work rather than comfort me, but I did feel good knowing that I would at least have one super-eye in the future.

'The left one ...' he paused for dramatic effect, '... that's even better than the right! Absolutely perfect. Your left eye is even stronger than the right.'

'Um, no it isn't,' I offered. 'I can't see a thing out the left eye.'

'Well, you should be able to because all the readings here say it is perfect. Spot on.'

Was Dr *Toeby Gyllan* trying to convince me I was wrong?

'Well, why can't I see anything through my left eye, then?' I asked.

'Your left eye, according to all my equipment and charts is perfect. I don't understand why you think there is a problem, Troy.'

'I don't think there is a problem, doc. I *know* there is a problem because I can't fucking see out of it!' I yelled.

'Okay, calm down. Let's try a few things. You may have distressed the eyeball when you rubbed it so it will take a few extra days to come good from your perspective. I can give you some special eye drops to use for a week, which will help to speed up the recovery. And in the right eye, keep using the eye drops you bought.'

'I haven't used the eye drops yet,' I told him.

A stunned silence fell over the room. If he had been holding a glass I'm sure he would have dropped it dramatically on the floor and passed out in a comical fashion at this announcement.

He spun on his heels and grabbed me by the shoulders.

'You *must* use the eye drops! Okay?'

'But my eyes aren't dry.'

'That doesn't matter. Your eyes *need* the eye drops. I cannot stress this enough. The drops are *essential*.'

I nodded, mostly out of fear, and promised to use the drops more than any man alive had ever used drops before. In the back of my mind, however, I was pretty sure I was lying.

The doctor's demeanour promptly returned to pleasant, as though the dire warnings of the previous moment had never occurred. He shook my hand and congratulated me on my successful surgery once more, despite my continual protesting, then sent me on my one-eyed way back into the world to wonder what I might look like with an eye-patch on.

It looks good on TV characters.

As it turns out, I wasn't lying about the eye drops, I simply didn't know it at the time. I had no intention of using the eye drops until about two days later when my eyes instantly felt like the Sahara Desert. Every blink felt like someone was running a nail file across my pupils and suddenly the makers of those eye drops became my greatest friends in the whole wide world.

Amazingly, the drops in my left eye eventually did make things come good. It took two months and three more free trips back to the eye clinic before I could finally see properly out of both eyes, and another three months after that before I could stop using the drops to keep my eyes moist. Stupid tear ducts!

These days my eyesight is perfect. I can see for miles and haven't owned a pair of glasses for years, which, oddly enough, no one has ever commented on.

It cost me $800, a few months of sleepless nights, a small fortune in eyedrops and gave me an inerasable memory of having my eyeballs rubbed with sandpaper while I watched on through taped-back eyelids ... and the weirdest part is, because I now have perfect eyesight, I'd do it all again in a heartbeat.

Luckily I'll never have to because that surgeon is no longer listed anywhere.

Or maybe he is — just under a different name.

# 16
# UP MY NOSE WITH a RUBBER HOSE

I've always liked the movie *Innerspace* with Martin Short and Dennis Quaid. I saw this film at the cinema in 1987, back when ticket prices were reasonable and you could actually afford to buy the popcorn as well. It's a comedy about a neurotic guy who has a miniature spaceship injected into his system, and it shows graphic footage of the inner workings of the human body.

As I was to discover, however, my insides look nothing like the movie version I saw on screen in the '80s. The film-makers made theirs with jelly moulds and cheap-looking special effects. Mine are a lot more confronting and disgusting. There's no way that Joe Dante's movie would ever have done as well as it did if they'd used real footage.

It was a year or two ago when I found myself with a weird sensation on the back, left side of my tongue. By 'weird', I mean it felt like there was something there. A bump, perhaps? Maybe a piece of old food? A splinter? Whatever it was, it didn't feel right.

As usual, I did nothing about it, other than complain loudly for a few weeks to my girlfriend and wish it would simply disappear. Then one day she'd grown even more frustrated by my illness than me and suggested I go and see a doctor about it. Seeing as I had thoroughly checked my tongue in the mirror over 200 times already and had discovered nothing in the vicinity of the irritation, I felt embarrassed about taking my invisible problem to a doctor, for fear that he'd think I was nuts. But my girlfriend had spoken and so I was on my way.

The doctor I saw at the medical centre that day agreed with my initial conclusion — that I was probably not of sound mind — but proceeded to shine all manner of torches into my mouth and make me say 'Ahhh' for what seemed like an eternity. Several times he placed a wooden stick onto my tongue to stop it moving around (and presumably to shut me up), and I wondered why they never thought of adding flavour to these implements. Every other time I'd had a wooden stick in my mouth, it was surrounded by ice-cream. That would certainly have been a more pleasant experience than this, and it would surely encourage more people to visit the doctor's surgery.

To any doctors out there, I'm giving you that idea for free. You'll double your number of patients and probably get a sponsorship deal with Streets. It's almost too good.

So, after discovering nothing with his torches and ice-cream-less wooden sticks, the doctor searched around in his desk for a few moments before uttering those words that no patient ever wants to hear: 'I'm going to refer you to a specialist.'

We all know what that means. In layman's terms it translates to: 'I know a guy who's missed a few mortgage payments on his holiday mansion. He could really use some of your hard-earned money.'

I have a theory that a doctor shouldn't charge you for your appointment if they refer you to a specialist. Basically, they didn't do anything or find anything wrong with you. All they've done is admit that they don't have the right qualifications and that you should probably go and see someone who does.

Of course, this doctor did charge me for his journey of non-discovery, then handed me a note that gave another, hopefully more qualified, individual permission to look at my invisible ailment as well. After paying my GP, begrudgingly, and leaving his office, I promptly phoned the number of the specialist whose details were on the note I'd been given.

'Hello, doctor's office,' said the woman on the other end of the phone.

'Ah, yes, hello. I have a referral here from my doctor to see Dr Hadden, if that's possible.'

'Well, Dr Hadden is retired so he only works on Wednesdays. Is next Wednesday okay for you?' she asked.

Retired? Firstly, if he was retired then why was he still working one day a week? And secondly, was it legal to practise medicine once you'd officially resigned from your profession? This all made me a little nervous.

'Sure, Wednesday would be fine,' I replied.

'Great, come in at about 1pm. Can I get your name, please?'

I ran through my details with her, hung up and began my wait until the following Wednesday, hoping that between now and then something might appear on my tongue to help me look less insane for Dr Hadden. It wasn't to be.

When the day finally came around, my tongue was as blemish-free and pink as it always had been. The weird sensation was still there, but given that I had nothing to show for it, I figured this meeting was never going to go very well. And I hate it when I'm right about that sort of thing.

I waited in Dr Hadden's reception area for only a few minutes before witnessing an elderly patient with a cane exit his office and shuffle slowly and painfully over to the reception desk. I felt bad for the old man, as I reflected that whatever reason he must've had for being here today might be truly debilitating and possibly bring about the end of his life. It was a sobering thought.

My feelings of sympathy were abruptly brought to a halt, however, when he turned from the desk with a piece of paper in his hand. 'Troy Harvey?' he asked.

My jaw dropped to the floor. 'Uh-huh ...' I nodded.

'Come in, come in. I'm Dr Hadden,' he said, turning unsteadily to shuffle back towards his office.

I rose from my chair and felt the need to steady him as he walked, much like a Cub Scout assisting a pensioner across a busy street. After a few moments of shuffling and teetering on his cane, Dr Hadden finally took a seat in his office, letting out an audible grunt as he did so.

This guy wasn't just old, he was clinically deceased. He must've retired some thirty years ago. So why was he still working on Wednesdays? Surely he should've been resting in a comfortable chair, eating liquid meals and occasionally complaining that the wireless in the nursing home was up too loud. Anything but working.

'So, what can we do for you today, Mr ...' He paused, trying to remember my name.

'Oh, Harvey!' I fired back.

'Yes — Mr O'Harvey. Hmm, they've left the O off your form here. I'll fix that.' He made a slow circle with his pen on my chart.

I didn't have the heart to correct him, as it had already taken five minutes to get from the hallway to his room. I figured my name was irrelevant to him anyway.

'Is that Irish?' he continued.

'Yes. My dad's Irish,' I lied.

'I see, I see. Now, what can we do for you today, son?'

'Well, it's kind of weird,' I began. 'I have this strange sensation on the back of my tongue, like there's a bump or something, but I can't see anything there. My doctor thought you should look at it.'

'Right then,' he responded with sudden excitement. 'Take a seat and we'll get a good look at it.'

I was already seated. I shuffled around in my chair for a few moments, wondering what to do next. Not wishing to hurt the poor man's feelings, I decided to raise myself slightly off the cushion and lower myself back down, just to act out the sitting process for Dr Hadden.

Meanwhile, he had managed to get up from his own chair and slowly make his way to my side. Here, he fiddled about with a small television screen that was on the shelf next to me and began to wipe down a long black cord that looked like it was the power lead.

'You'll need this,' he commented, handing over a small bottle of nasal spray.

'What for?'

'Spray some up your right nostril for me. It'll numb the area.'

Again I felt the need to query the old man. 'What for?' I repeated.

'It makes it less uncomfortable when I insert the camera,' he answered mysteriously.

At this point I noticed that the cord he was cleaning was connected to the TV at one end, but completely without the electrical prongs you'd normally find at the other. Was he really going to stick that thing up my nose? Didn't I make it clear that the problem was with my tongue? Even I could see my tongue from the front. Why would he need to go in from the top?

'Er, it's my tongue that's the problem,' I mumbled.

'Yes, but we'll need to see if there's anything else there or down the back of your throat, in order to be sure it isn't something more serious,' he replied. 'Don't worry, son. Just relax.'

Those words made me shudder. Not wanting to think about my impending nasal invasion, I placed the spray into my nose and began pumping furiously to numb the region. I didn't want to feel one second of this.

'That's enough, that's enough,' said Dr Hadden, prying the bottle from my clenched fist. 'Now, put your head back and try to breathe normally.'

As he spoke these words, he forcefully jammed a black rubber tube into my left nostril. That's right, my *left*. Keen observers will recall that he told me to numb the right-hand nostril. Dr Hadden had obviously meant his right, not mine. Brilliant.

I spluttered like a drowning victim as the cable made its way awkwardly through the back of my nose and started to worry that it was touching my brain, until I felt it graze the back of my throat, making me gag loudly.

'That's a good boy. Gooooood boy,' cooed Dr Hadden, patting me on the head.

Was this guy once a vet? I hoped he wasn't planning to take my temperature at any stage.

'Keep breathing. Good boy. Very good boy.'

It was incredibly awkward. He was patting my head like you would a distressed pet. I almost expected him to hand me a snack as a treat.

'Have a look here on the screen for a moment, son,' he said as I struggled for air.

Weirdly enough, I had completely neglected to look at the TV since the start of this ordeal. It was just out of my peripheral vision, and up until now I'd only been thinking of ways to escape.

Glancing sideways, I was greeted with one of the most disgusting pictures I have ever seen on a TV screen. It was live coverage of my throat and, had I stared at it for a fraction of a second longer, we would probably have also seen live coverage of projectile vomit making its way past the camera on its way to my specialist's shoes. I looked away, gagged violently again and suppressed my urge to hurl.

'Just relax. Good boy. Gooood boy,' continued Dr Hadden as he began sliding the tube slowly out of my nose and onto the side bench.

It was truly horrendous. But with the unpleasant part now over, the old man started out on the return trip back to his desk.

'Well, nothing there to worry about, son,' he offered in his grandfatherly fashion.

'You mean, there's nothing in my throat?' I spluttered, still wiping my mouth and nose with the tissue he'd given me.

'Nothing at all. Seems your tongue is probably rubbing against your tooth at night. That can happen sometimes. Might be bad dreams. Do you have bad dreams, son?'

'I will now,' I said honestly.

'Well, you need to avoid stress in your days and try to eat well at night. That usually helps.'

Never showing me that camera view of my throat would've helped as well, I imagined.

'You'll be fine,' he added. 'Is there anything else I can help you with?'

'Er, no, that's all. Thank you,' I said and showed myself out before Dr Hadden could even lift himself out of his chair.

The receptionist stared at me blankly for a few seconds and then handed me a tissue from her desk. Obviously I still had liquids dripping off my face, but I assumed she'd see that every Wednesday, when Dr Hadden came in to treat his patients. I simply wiped my nose and handed over my credit card in response.

By the sound the machine made when she swiped the card, I could tell my savings had taken a beating. Her eyes lit up slightly as well. All up, this little adventure ended up costing me over

$200 to discover that, as usual, whatever condition I thought I had was actually nothing. And that it would, as usual, heal itself a few weeks later.

So next time you're sitting in a cinema, complaining about the high ticket prices and average special effects, just remember that it could be a lot worse. You could be watching real life instead — and paying a couple of hundred bucks for the privilege.

# 17
# AFTER BURN: THE BURNING CONCLUSION

'It's your back, mate,' said Dr Tessler, matter-of-factly describing the cause for the burning sensation in my thighs and groin.

'What? No, it's my front,' I explained for what felt like the one-thousandth time.

'I know that's where it's manifesting the pain, but trust me — it's caused by your back. And I can prove it,' he continued, raising an eyebrow.

This guy was good. I'd come to Dr Tessler after so many other doctors had failed me in the past. Yet he was simply the closest medical practitioner to my new place of work. I'd visited him one day after the burning sensation had flared up again, so he was now the keeper of the flame, so to speak.

After telling him the same old story and begging for assistance, he had sensibly conducted every test under the sun and shown me once again in black-and-white that not only did I not have any of the diseases I'd once convinced myself I had, but also that I was the healthiest man alive. This was good news indeed — bordering on the 'Testes, 100 per cent' level of good news.

Of course, that still didn't explain why my groin occasionally experienced a painful burning sensation. But Dr Tessler could.

'Your x-rays came back and I looked at them before you got here,' he informed me.

He'd made me get x-rays on my back a few days earlier. Normally I would have told him he was insane and wasting my time, but by this stage I was tired of fighting with doctors and pretty much open to any suggestion. Strangely enough, this suggestion would turn out to be the best I'd ever heard.

'Take a look here, mate.' Dr Tessler was pointing at an x-ray of my spine, which he then replaced with an MRI scan of the same general vicinity.

'Hmmm,' I hummed, not wanting to look stupid even though I had no idea what he was pointing at.

'You have a crack in one of your lower discs,' he said.

'Oh dear!' To be honest, I was still confused as to how this related to my groin.

'Relax — it's okay. It's not the worst news in the world. It means that it's occasionally trapping your nerve.'

'I see ...' My blank expression was totally giving me away.

'Listen — you have nerves in your spine. They come down and radiate out into your body. Down here, they radiate to your groin and thighs. It's called the pudendal nerve and when it gets trapped, you feel the pain down at the nerve endings. Do you understand?'

Oddly enough, I did. And even more oddly enough, it made sense.

'So, you're saying I've got a couple of trapped nerves? *That's* what's caused all this pain and anguish?'

'Yep.'

'Are you sure?' I asked, desperate for a definitive answer.

'Yep. Absolutely. It's right there on the screen, mate. Think about it, whenever you've had the nerve trapped, you've thought it was something more serious, tensed up and become stressed — which has only gone and made it worse. Then, when you've been told it's not something scary, you've relaxed and it's fixed itself. Do you not understand how simple this is?'

'But how do you explain the fact that all this started after I kissed a girl?' I asked, trying to complete the puzzle.

'It has nothing to do with the girl, mate. That's just what you recall from the time because you thought you'd caught something. It's more likely that you trapped a nerve by lifting your luggage when you went on your holiday. Or sitting in an airplane seat for an hour or two. Either of those makes more sense than your ridiculous theory.'

I wanted to hug him. 'So how do I fix it?' I enquired with some apprehension.

'Well, we can cut a small hole in your back ...'

Instantly reminded of my earlier back-cutting incident, I recoiled in horror. Fortunately for me, Dr Tessler had a second option.

'Or, you could take a bucket-load of muscle relaxants and it'll probably go away. Personally, I'd smash down a whole packet of them over a couple of days and you should be fine.'

'And that's it?' I asked, astonished.

'That's it. Other than that, you're ridiculously healthy. So stop going on the internet and self-diagnosing. No good can come from it. We've done every test you can do, and I've proved conclusively that you don't have any diseases or problems whatsoever. Get over it.'

It was pretty sensible advice, although that didn't stop me pushing the point too far. 'But the internet knows everything!' I yelled in the World Wide Web's defence.

'Mate, the web is full of viruses, hackers, thieves, pornographers, scammers and other criminals. What could possibly make you think the medical information on there is any better?'

Touché.

'You're *fine!*' he told me loudly and clearly. 'Completely healthy. You don't have anything other than a trapped nerve. Nothing else — believe me, I've checked several times over. Now, come back when you actually have something to show me!'

It was nice to hear. I mean, that's what we all really want to hear in life — that we're doing okay — isn't it?

And so with that glorious announcement and a handful of muscle relaxants, that was it. My pain went away and it has never come back since. I'm as healthy as a horse.

To be honest, I still can't understand how all the intricate parts of the body work together so perfectly, but I'm sure glad they do. And for as long as they do, I should probably be pretty grateful.

So the next time I wake up and something, somewhere, on my body hurts, burns, itches or bursts, maybe I'll just stop for a moment, relax, and assume that everything's going to be okay.

Well, at least until my girlfriend tells me I should go and see a doctor about it, anyway.

# 18
# SO, WHAT CAN BE LEARNED FROM ALL THIS?

I believe every experience in life is a learning experience, and it helps to remind myself of this every time I recall the hundreds of hours and thousand of dollars I've wasted on trying to cure ailments and injuries that have mostly gone on to cure themselves.

So, with *your* health and hip pocket in mind, here's some advice I can give to all the men out there who don't want to go through the hell I've been through over the past decade or so.

+ A burning sensation on or around the penis might not be an STD. It may just mean someone is talking about it.

+ If you're having a heart attack, don't drive yourself anywhere. It's a pretty stupid thing to do. On the other hand, if you're *not* having a heart attack, maybe drive around for a while and keep an eye out for someone who is.

✤ Doctors don't seem to mind looking up your bum, so don't be shy when asking them to. Friends, on the other hand, do mind. Don't ask them.

✤ If you have to buy a cream for an embarrassing ailment, the name of that cream will always be twice as embarrassing as the ailment was in the first place. Don't buy it.

✤ Hypnotherapy doesn't involve capes, sequins, dangling watches or a beautiful assistant. It is a spectacular disappointment. Avoid it.

✤ The most ominous words you will ever hear from a doctor are: 'Just relax.' When you hear those words, don't relax — something bad is about to happen.

✤ Googling your symptoms for a diagnosis is the worst thing you can ever do for your blood pressure. According to my internet searches, I've had everything from vaginal itching and feline rickets to spontaneous human combustion. Don't trust the web.

✤ If everybody leaves the room so that a machine can begin scanning you, that machine is doing more than scanning you. Try to protect your sperm.

✤ Optometrists need to get up close to your face. Very close. They're not trying to make out with you, though, so don't mistake an eye test for a romantic gesture.

✤ The physio is far and away the coolest person a man can ever pretend to visit. Make an appointment. You don't even have to go.

✤ Stressing about a condition, before you know what that condition actually is, can sometimes lead to another condition appearing, purely because you hoped it wouldn't. The human body is fucked up like that.

✤ Don't make fun of humourless doctors, mid-surgery. They don't like it.

✤ Iran *does* have acupuncturists. Don't be so racist.

✤ No matter how much you beg, no medical professional will ever let you officially name your yet-to-be-discovered condition 'The Roasted Nuts of Troy Harvey'. But ask anyway.

✤ Listen to women when they tell you to go and visit a doctor. You don't actually have a choice, and if it turns out to be something serious and you never went, they'll get to say 'I told you so' for the rest of your life ... which may end up being a lot shorter because you never did what they said.

✤ Don't always listen to your doctor when they claim to know what might be wrong with you. Ask them for proof.

But most importantly of all: try to laugh. There's a reason that millions of jokes start with the line 'A man walks into a doctor's office ...'

One day we'll all be told that whatever it is we're experiencing health-wise will lead us to an untimely death (not that I've ever heard of a *timely* one, mind you). So, until that day, whatever doesn't kill you may indeed make you stronger. Or, at the very least, it may lead you to receive a piece of paper that confirms, beyond a shadow of a doubt, that your testicles are 100 per cent. And, guys, isn't that what we're all really striving for in this world?

Of course it is.

So, to give you all something to aspire to during your limited time here on earth, I present to you now my plums of perfection:

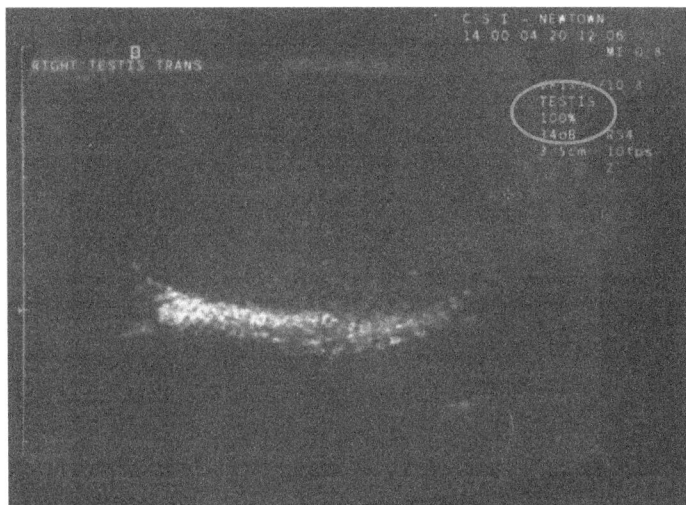

# acknowledgments

This book would never have seen the light of day without the love and encouragement of my beautiful partner Elizabeth, who believed in me even when it seemed as though everyone else, including myself, had lost faith. I adore you.

I would like to offer a never-ending stream of gratitude to everyone at HarperCollins, with special mention of thanks to Sandy Weir, Julian Gray and Anne Reilly, who put up with all my rambling phone calls. Your support, endless patience and extraordinary levels of kindness are greatly appreciated. Thank you to Jon Gibbs for helping to craft my crazed rants so well.

I'd also like to thank every medical professional who ever treated me and managed to keep a straight face. Your names have been changed in this book to protect the innocent (and by 'the innocent' I mean: me from lawsuits), but you probably know who you are.

For always making me laugh, no matter what I was going through, I wish to thank Tony Martin, Jon Stewart, Shaun Micallef and Working Dog.

And most importantly, thank you to my wonderful and supportive family who, for reasons known only to themselves, still haven't disowned me. You are the greatest people I know.

www.ingramcontent.com/pod-product-compliance
Lightning Source LLC
Chambersburg PA
CBHW032139020426
42334CB00016B/1216